WASSON

PHYSICAL THERAPY AND MASSAGE FOR THE HORSE

Jean-Marie Denoix

Professor,
École Nationale Vétérinaire, Alfort

Jean-Pierre Pailloux

Physiotherapist to the
French National Equestrian Team 1986–88 and
at the Seoul Olympics

Translated by
Jonathan Lewis

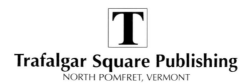

Trafalgar Square Publishing
NORTH POMFRET, VERMONT

Reprinted 1997
**First published in the United States of America in 1996 by
Trafalgar Square Publishing, North Pomfret, Vermont 05053
ISBN: 1-57076-021-7**

Library of Congress Catalog Card Number: 94–61970

Printed and bound by Dah Hua Printing Press Co., Hong Kong.

Copyright © Manson Publishing Ltd 1996

First published in France in 1989 by Éditions Maloine

Typeset and designed by Paul Bennett, Tonbridge, Kent, England.

Contents

Preface

Competition in equine sports is becoming increasingly intense.

It is perhaps time for all of us who are involved to set aside highly artificial techniques and concentrate on what is essential - the quality of preparation and aftercare.

Our aim should be to produce movement which is natural and joyous and rewarding both for the horse and for ourselves.

Human athletes have no problem in discussing their concerns about performance or injury. Their equine counterparts, required to submit to commands and unable to communicate, are, however, not so fortunate. In a context where the only voices heard and priorities established are our own, the horse is frequently misunderstood. We should not be surprised if impaired performance is the result.

Physiotherapy is based on the understanding of and respect for biomechanical structures. It has already made a considerable contribution to human athletic endurance and performance. It is, however, more than just a therapeutic technique: through touch and gesture it is also a means of sensory communication, of bridging the silence between horse and rider.

This book, the product of the collaboration between an experienced equestrian and a physiotherapist, has been written with the purpose of explaining the new approaches to the care of the horse that physiotherapy offers and the role that it can play in developing the potential of the equine athlete, from the moment that the foal takes its first steps.

I owe a special debt to Professor Jean-Marie Denoix, whose observations, precise anatomical descriptions and richly detailed drawings have been so important to the realization of this book.

Jean-Pierre Pailloux

PART ONE

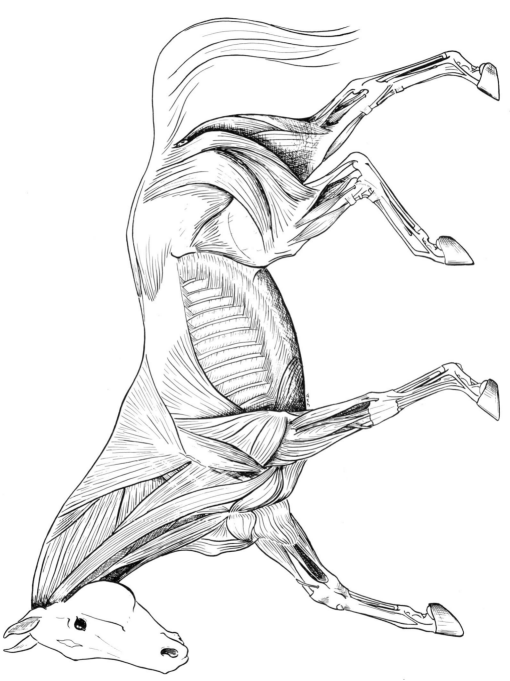

Figure 1 Superficial musculature of the Horse.

1 Concepts of Neuromuscular Physiology

The majority of medicines are the product of observation, empiricism and analogy. In Ancient Egypt and in the Graeco-Roman world, no distinction was made between human and animal medicines. Melanpos, a shepherd and doctor who is mentioned in Virgil, used the same potions when treating the daughters of King Argos and animals. Theomneste used an ointment which contained 31 ingredients to treat both men and horses. Healers applied their knowledge to men and animals alike.

Physiotherapy continues this empirical approach, but within the context of modern science; its practice stretches back to Antiquity, but it applies present-day standards of mathematical precision to massage, electrotherapy and physiology.

Today's medical or veterinary student depends more on his or her memory of scientific fact than on instinct. However, therapy itself often involves appreciable mathematical precision; the practice of healing, which is the product of thousands of years of observation and treatment, has adjusted to the advances of modern therapeutic techniques.

Physiotherapy provides solutions to a variety of preventive and therapeutic situations in human medicine. It has already proven its effectiveness in its application to sport, where much progress has been made due to the the pooling of knowledge by researchers, doctors and physiotherapists. It should therefore help develop new approaches to the treatment of the horse.

Many young people coming into veterinary science are interested in new ideas, and are frustrated with the old-fashioned dualistic approach which places science and therapy in separate compartments. It is important to offer them encouragement, developing their creativity without dampening their enthusiasm. Dialogue between veterinarians and physiotherapists must become as open as that between the various specialties in human medicine.

The career of an athlete, whether man or horse, requires talent, hard work, a methodical approach and the provision of a prophylactic and therapeutic medical environment. Equine sports medicine is well established, but it is still relatively new and must develop further in order to provide an appropriate level of support for equestrian sports. Physiotherapy treats the muscles involved in sport, and is thus central to this process.

The movement and locomotion of the horse, and the improvement and maintenance of performance, are the subject of constant observation and concern. However, these should not focus on the mechanical aspects alone. Locomotion does not occur independently of the neuro-regulatory system, which has a direct influence on the strength or weakness of a particular action and is the source of positive or inhibitory neuromotive impulses.

A favourable psychological and neuro-regulatory environment provides a healthy and nurturing dynamic; conversely, the first signs of illness or distress can often be detected in poorly coordinated and precipitate movements.

Physiotherapy and biomechanics are concerned with the study of the following aspects of the horse:

1. NEUROPHYSIOLOGY

1.1 THE BRAIN'S LIMBIC SYSTEM

The limbic lobe, discovered by Broca in 1878, is a convolution that surrounds the brain stem. While an evolutionary legacy of reptilian characteristics is evident, the lobe is endowed with a more advanced section which is free of the stereotypical behaviour of the more primitive part of the brain. As with all of the higher vertebrates, one of its essential functions is the detection of unusual, new or unexpected phenomena.

In mammals the limbic system is above all responsible for emotional behaviour, generating active or passive responses appropriate to the situation. It is the source of emotional expression and anxiety, but also the area where logic and confidence are developed.

The horse, always on its guard, timid and lacking courage, must be approached and supervised with care. Some riders manage better than others in this respect. The horse's essential nature cannot be changed, and the potential of very promising horses can be ruined because they are anxious and not understood.

With the emotional aspect so dominant, the judicious rider will recognize the need for a calm and confident approach. The importance of communication between horse and rider is obvious, as is the nervousness that characterises some horse-rider relationships.

1.2 ANXIETY AND MUSCULAR TONUS

The horse's muscles provide the earliest indications of anxiety. Muscular tonus is closely involved with variations in in its psychological state. It is important to recognize that emotional equilibrium is as vital to optimum sporting performance as the physiological readiness of the underlying mechanical structures, which will not perform on command unless the horse is comfortable and confident. Tonus, posture and locomotion are closely linked to muscular contraction.

Definition of tonus: its implications for the relationship between horse and rider

Tonus is the light contractile tension which informs and surrounds every skeletal muscle which is not directly involved in a specific activity and is at rest. Basic tonus is the state of awareness that maintains the horse's posture while it is at rest, in a state of psychological and physiological comfort and not being subjected to any kind of emotional disturbance. Tonus changes when it is subjected to two kinds of influence:

External
- Aggressive behaviour within the horse's immediate environment, producing hypertonia.
- A peaceful environment, which promotes basic tonus.
- Medication which, according to the drug administered, can produce either hypertonia or hypotonia, or a return to basic tonus.

Internal
(a) Psychological
- Aggressiveness, producing an increase in tonus.
- Fatigue, producing a decrease (sometimes an increase) in tonus.
- Fear, stress, anxiety, competition, producing an increase (sometimes a decrease) in tonus.
(b) Pathological
- Illness, fatigue: producing an increase or decrease in tonus.

Disorders due to variations in tonus can be found in and interpreted from the horse's performance. The ideal sporting action occurs in a positive frame of mind and psychological well-being. In the rider, competition can generate a level of anxiety that can be detected by the horse and add to its own level of stress. Signs of the horse's nervousness manifest at the muscular level in an increase in tonus, which can, if well managed – and provided that opposing muscle groups do not become rigid – improve performance. Methods of developing a closer correspondence between the tonus of horse and rider include:

1. Awareness of the relative levels of tonus.
2. Focusing on the points of tension:
- Rider: relaxation of hands and thighs, suppleness in back and shoulders;
- Horse: looseness of the back, with freedom of lateral and neck movement.
3. Modifying the training schedule in accordance with observation, with light stimulation to treat hypotonus and lengthy periods of relaxation to help calm nervousness.

This will help control superfluous and non-productive nervous activity in both horse and rider. Recreational activities can also be employed.

1.3 THE DEVELOPMENT OF SPATIAL COGNITION AND PROPRIOCEPTION

Boris Dolto[1] has observed that the development of spatial cognition and proprioception in both man and horse proceeds in stages, from birth until the point at which the body is perceived to function separately from the external world. The foal becomes aware of its body by looking at it and from contact with objects in its immediate environment. Spatial coordination proceeds gradually, eventually leading to skill in movement. Development in the horse is more rapid than in man due to psychomotor ability being much more advanced at birth – the foal is able to walk immediately – and also to a lesser dependence on the mother. The major areas of the body most frequently used to acquire sensory information include:

1. The upper lip, which is richly innervated, hence the inhibitory action of twitching.
2. The forelegs, which the horse is aware of at an early stage, and which are used frequently in deliberate movements such as pawing, stamping and playing with objects.

[1] B. Dolto. *Le corps entre les mains*. Une nouvelle kinésithérapie. Herman.

The hind legs and vertebral column, which are removed from the foal's immediate field of vision, are the sources of unknown – and to the foal inexplicable – physical sensations, and thus adjust more slowly in the development of awareness. The weight of a rider, back tension or pain can further retard the process.

Accidents affect proprioception. The sensation of pain in a limb can disturb and frighten the horse, causing it to move clumsily. The process of reeducation, once movement is no longer painful, is slow. Recovery following an accident in a sporting event must be allowed to proceed gradually. Riders frequently make no allowance for a lack of coordination during the period of recuperation, becoming demanding and thus creating indelibly disturbing impressions in the horse's mind. This can cause:

1. Loss of coordination during obstacle jumping or dressage.
2. Anxiety, over-excitability, inhibition, impaired performance and loss of commitment.

1.4 PROPRIOCEPTORS AND THE SENSORIMOTOR SYSTEM

(a) Proprioceptors and the processing of information

The proprioceptors (position sensory receptors) are situated in the ligaments, tendons, muscles and joints, and provide the information required to adjust posture and movement (Fig. 2). They influence the responses required to correct imbalance due to muscular or ligamentary tension caused by a badly placed or twisted foot, or an unforeseen stretching movement. The centres in the spinal cord and brain are made aware of a situation and respond accordingly. For example, when a foot loses contact with the ground on encountering a hole, it is retracted immediately.

After an accident, proprioception is modified by the new sensations of pain and lameness. The body progressively organizes itself to cope with these biodynamic messages by adjusting its behaviour. It attempts to avoid the experience of further pain either by limiting movement of the joint, or by compensating for it through using other muscles, sometimes a combination of the two.

Therapy must take these facts into account. It must go beyond immediate attention to a lesion by envisaging the treatment required for muscles at some distance from it which are compensating for the skeletal muscles flinching as a result of the pain (for example, a reflex paravertebral contraction caused by a lesion in the leg).

Moreover, a horse which has regained soundness of movement will continue to retain for several weeks a vivid memory of its distress. It will move gingerly, out of apprehension that its movements will still be painful. The convalescing horse must be allowed to recover and have its confidence restored by a closely supervised programme of exercise, otherwise the image of the trauma will be retained.

(b) Neuromotive reaction

Information issuing from the proprioceptors deep in the cybernetic muscles, ligaments and tendons is analysed for tensions or stretching movements (Fig. 3). Following on from this analysis, instructions are given to correct posture or muscular tonus and regain orthopaedic equilibrium.

A horse leaving its box after a long period of inactivity will emerge with its neurosensory centres basically 'awake', but will find its locomotion hampered by a lack of postural information and overall tonus. Physiological adaptation to the movement that is now required is extensive and proceeds in stages; it involves stretching of the fetlock or pastern joints,

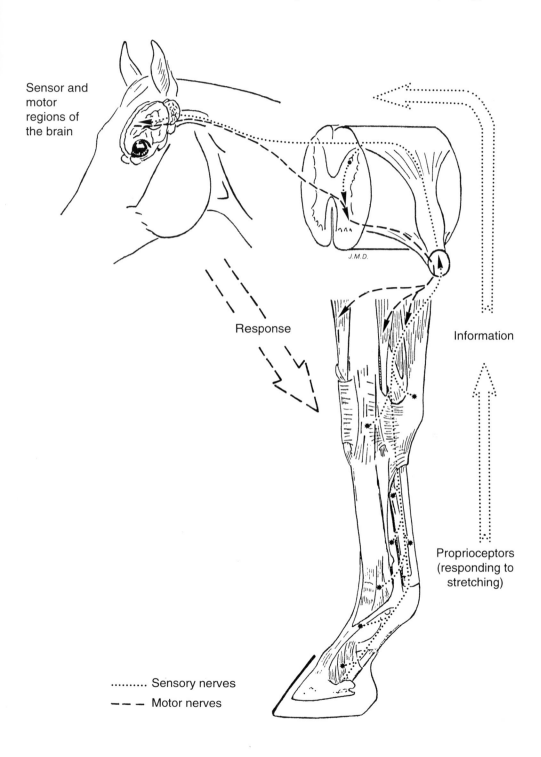

Sensor and
motor
regions of
the brain

Response

Information

Proprioceptors
(responding to
stretching)

.... Sensory nerves

‒ ‒ ‒ Motor nerves

J.M.D.

Figure 2 Regulation of muscular tension by stretching the tendons and
ligaments.

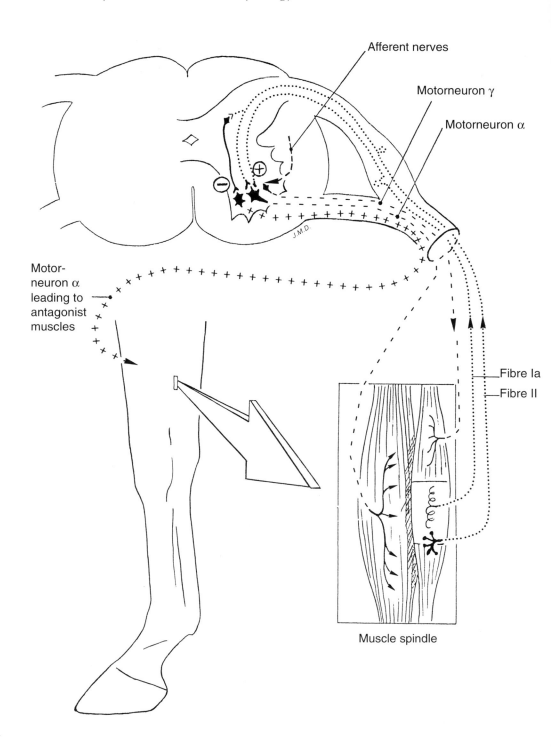

Figure 3 Feedback loop.

contraction of the muscles and elongation of the ligaments. The neuromotive reaction is influenced by a number of factors, including type of horse, morphology, weight, age and general condition. Consideration of these factors induces a respect for the horse's physiology and the way it adapts itself to effort.

(c) Factors affecting muscular response

Perception of, and the rapidity of response to, information depend on the speed of conductivity within the nervous system (Fig. 4). The following factors can affect the speed and effectiveness with which postural imbalance is corrected following a sudden, unforeseen stretching of a muscle or ligament:

Positive factors
1. Good quality bloodline.
2. Lightness of weight.
3. Maturity: the adult horse possesses a fully developed mechanism of response and control.
4. Genetic origin: Arabs, Berbers and American ponies are accustomed to a variety of hard, gravelly and mountainous terrain, which is excellent for developing proprioception.

Negative factors
1. Poor quality bloodline.
2. Heaviness: weight on the joints is increased, making injury more likely.
3. Age: with time the horse loses its proprioceptive ability.

2. DEVELOPMENT AND ADAPTATION OF NEUROPHYSIOLOGICAL RESPONSE

The various factors which condition neuromuscular physiology are neither static nor definitive, but evolve over time as a response to training and according to the individual horse's state of health.

2.1 NEUROMOTOR REHABILITATION FOLLOWING INJURY

Proprioceptive re-education contributes to the recovery of coordination, thereby becoming a form of neuromotor rehabilitation. The proprioception of injured horses is adapted to mitigate pain. As painless, easy, movements are replaced by unfamiliar sensations – pain, lameness and imbalance – the horse's usual behaviour is inhibited. There are many examples of horses which are unable to recover fully. For this reason, proprioceptive re-education, which restores positive reinforcement messages and helps the horse to return to its former level of performance, is invaluable.

There are two methods for achieving this. The first involves letting the horse run on a number of differing natural terrains, creating a variety of plantar sensations and movements.

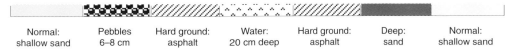

| Normal:
shallow sand | Pebbles
6–8 cm | Hard ground:
asphalt | Water:
20 cm deep | Hard ground:
asphalt | Deep:
sand | Normal:
shallow sand |

Figure 4 Sensory re-education path. Each section is between 3 and 6 metres in length, which is sufficient to allow the horse to adapt to each new sensation.

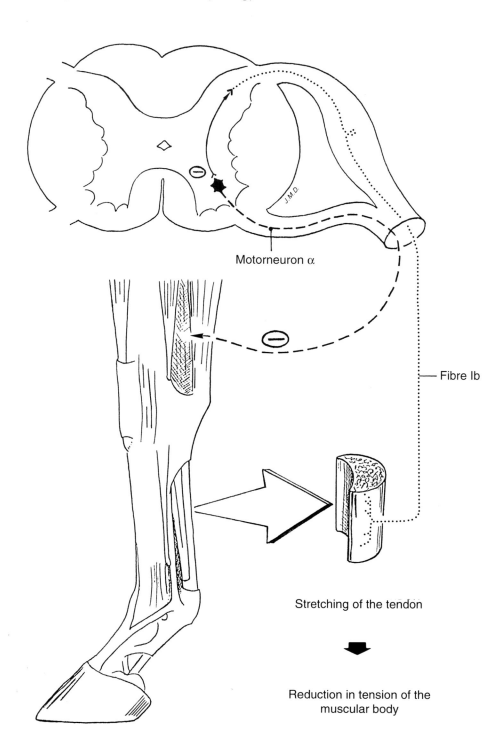

Motorneuron α

Fibre Ib

Stretching of the tendon

Reduction in tension of the
muscular body

Figure 5 Golgi receptors.

The second involves the creation of an artificial path, termed the sensory re-education path (henceforth SRP) (Fig. 4), where the horse encounters a number of terrains in sequence. The latter method facilitates more rapid progress because it allows for closer supervision and a greater variety of stimulation. Surfaces varying in depth and hardness are placed close to each other. As the horse encounters each section (which is 3 to 6 metres long), the differing consistency – deep and shallow sand, hard asphalt, pebbles and water – causes it to adapt rapidly. The process enhances the rapidity of response and functioning of the neuroreceptors. The stimuli are stored within the horse's memory and eventually lead to soundness of movement.

(a) SRP protocol

It is advisable to start the series of exercises as soon as the horse is no longer lame. The horse is gently led along the SRP, and allowed to see where it is placing its feet.

Duration: on the first day, three minutes on each rein, at a walk. This should increase progressively by a minute on each subsequent day. By the end of the recuperation period, the exercise should last for up to 15 minutes. It is neither logical nor efficient to try to rehabilitate a joint while neglecting the whole complex area of perception and control.

In human medicine, similar methods of sensory and proprioceptive education have been instrumental in reducing the need for plastic surgery by 50%.

2.2 PREPARATORY STRETCHING AND SUPPLING EXERCISES

When supervised and and programmed, stretching can enhance the awareness of the proprioceptors. 'Awakening' them in this way is therapeutic and prepares the horse for immediate action. Stretching can be either passive – administered to the horse while it is still in its box – or active.

Stretching is of fundamental importance, as it brings the proprioceptors in the ligaments and tendons to a state of readiness. It improves balance and frees up movement, without risking premature effort from muscles which are in an inappropriate state of tonus. In the absence of preliminary stretching, putting the horse to work too abruptly can bring on the following:

1. Dorsolumbar cramps.
2. Reflex muscle contractions caused by the back being 'cold'; instead of the spine engaging the hind legs, the extensor muscles stiffen and lock up.

The intensity of effort involved in activities such as jumping and trot extensions is dependent on:

1. Readiness of the proprioceptors involved in postural balance and defensive reflex actions.
2. Triggering of the reflexes that coordinate movement.
3. Preparation of the horse so that it is at an appropriate level of tonus.

Neglecting to provide an adequate preparatory regime is common practice, and is either the result of overtraining or due to simple indifference to the rules which govern biomechanical health. It is not unusual to see a horse, which has been in a box for 24 hours, put to three laps at the canter on each rein before immediately commencing its first jumps. Attention to preparation of the muscles and ligaments prior to performance allows both young and older horses alike to adapt and regulate the physiological vertebral system. It develops freedom of movement in the back, neck and lateral muscles involved in the lengthening of the spinal column. One exercise involves drawing the nose of the horse in lateral and downwards movements in opposition to the normal lateral movements of the trunk. It should be practised at each of the three gaits.

2.3 PROGRESS IN PERFORMANCE

(a) Development of sensitivity

Neuromotive and intuitive influences can be detected in the gestural language of the horse and accentuate the need for the development of sensitivity and communication between horse and rider. Without sensitivity and finesse – the features that distinguish the experienced rider from the beginner – there can be no horsemanship. Physiologically, the development from the unschooled gait of the foal, which can be heavy and imprecise, to the acquisition of coordinated impulsion is achieved during the course of an apprenticeship, in which the horse is trained to memorize simple and carefully thought out commands. Analysis of these commands shows that both the rider's intentions and the horse's perception of and reaction to them must be taken into account.

From the time of Xenophon (5th century BC) to the School of Versailles and on down to the present day, there have been many proponents of the light-handed approach. However, present-day schools, in their desire to keep up with the demands of competition, frequently neglect to practise it. As physical activity becomes more intense, openness and communication between rider and horse correspondingly suffer. The good results achieved by women riders at the highest levels of competition, and in all the disciplines, emphasize the importance of the horse/rider relationhip. Conrad Homfeld has underlined the existence of the two contrasting attitudes – feminine sensitivity and masculine firmness. G. Morris, in a recent work dealing with communication, has also dealt with this subject.

Proficient performance, for human and equine athlete alike, is achieved gradually. Over time, clumsy and gauche movements become controlled and coordinated. They are 'tamed' by neurophysiological development and by the diversification of muscular roles, which together gradually imprint within the horse's memory the appropriate articular action. Taking the concert hall as an analogy, the less noise there is within the hall, the easier it is to hear the different instruments in the orchestra. This diversification, as Boris Dolto has put it with his customary clarity, involves distinguishing the 'gymnastic' from the 'cybernetic' muscles. These roles complement each other, but also allow a measure of individuality. They lie behind the preparation for successful competitive performance. At this point, it is worth emphasizing two principles essential to the well thought-out training programme:

1. Adaptation through exercise of the prominent muscle groups involved in impulsion.
2. Development of the horse's sensory and proprioceptive musculature, to a level at which it will respond to the least pressure from the rider.

The young horse's progress from basic to sensitive movement should be envisaged in terms of a training programme in which the 'alphabet' initially consists of large letters and in which the focus is on muscular relationships. Once a measure of control of locomotion and posture has been achieved, the focus shifts to the reinforcement of the message of restraint in movement. Steinbrecht discusses this aspect in his *Horse's Training School*[1].

[1] G. Steinbrecht. *Le gymnase du cheval*. 4e édition, 1935. Editions Elbé.

As the apprenticeship proceeds, the trainer adapts the simple and dynamic commands appropriate to the young horse, which become less purely physical and accompanied by aids of various kinds, and more sensitive. The 'alphabet' becomes successively refined. Economy of muscular and articular movement, together with steadiness of behaviour, become permanent when forceful command is replaced by communication, and help prepare the horse for a future of restrained, heathy and pain-free impulsion.

Once the sensory aspect becomes dominant, the purely physical becomes less so. It is its ability to interpret (through its sensitive 'cybernetic' muscles) the variety of pressures and gestures applied by the rider that allows the horse to assess the latter's wishes and perform appropriately. In order to develop an increasingly subtle level of communication, it is important to ensure that the horse is not distressed, tired or in pain. It will then show its pleasure with a committed and vibrant performance. This exchange can lead to an almost uncanny level of communication when great artistic talent is involved, with horse and rider losing themselves in the intensity of their dialogue.

(b) Differentiation between cybernetic and gymnastic muscles

The gymnastic muscles are the most important and strongest skeletal muscles, responsible for rapidity and power of impulsion. Their innervation is relatively light, with one motorneuron servicing approximately 1000 myofibrils.

The cybernetic muscles, by contrast, are richly innervated (with one neuron servicing 20 to 30 myofibrils), which makes their movement much more precise. Examples include the muscles in the upper lip and the orbicular muscle in the eyelids, with one neuron for each two muscle fibres. These sensitive muscles are also located deep in the body, in the regions next to articular joints (notably around the spinal column), and are in contact with the capsular and ligamentary membranes. Proprioceptors transmit information on the muscles' state of tension to the brain via reflex paths. Their proximity to the joints, the wealth of postural information they contain and the variety of possible responses which they are capable of are the features which distinguish them from the gymnastic muscles. It is the cybernetic muscles which respond to the rider's subtler commands.

These proprioceptive muscles have a particular role to play in the development of sensitivity. For them to be effective the horse must be attuned:

1. *Psychologically:* if the horse is stressed, the gymnastic muscles can take over to the extent that proprioceptive awareness is obscured, locking the muscles and joints.
2. *Physiologically:* if illness or pain or some mechanical restriction hampers soundness of movement, the horse's perceptions and responses, and particularly its proprioception, can be adversely affected.

Conflict between the two kinds of muscle occurs in certain situations, such as when a young horse is tired or being verbally harassed and handled brusquely. As a rule, if there is a well-balanced relationship between horse and rider, gymnastic and cybernetic muscles complement each other. If psychological and physiological communication is poor – and the aware rider is as much a psychologist as a physiotherapist – the work will suffer accordingly, and the horse's future successful performance will be hampered.

(c) Attention to muscular fatigue

Many miles of work imposed on the young horse, without breaks, rest and appropriate preparation, will totally block the neurosensory system, with the main muscle groups becoming spasmodic and painful. Finesse of movement cannot co-exist with overwork. The horse is not mindlessly altruistic, a machine which builds muscle simply in order to compete. It should be seen as an acrobat endowed with harmony of movement. A tightrope walker is not expected to perform artistically after intense muscular effort, when his movements are likely to uncontrolled and trembling from fatigue, and neither is the horse. The following diagram illustrates the principles discussed in this chapter.

ATTENTION TO MUSCULAR FATIGUE
MAKING THE GYMNASTIC ASPECT OF PERFORMANCE LESS DOMINANT
ARE CENTRAL TO
PROGRESSIVE BIODYNAMIC DEVELOPMENT
AND COORDINATED IMPULSION

NEUROSENSORY PERCEPTION which leads to NEURSENSORY MEMORIZATION

 Development of spatial cognition and proprioception
Development of sensitivity
Maintenance of soundness
Commitment and reciprocity from the horse

(d) Respect for the horse's age and rate of progress

It is important to give the young horse plenty of space and time in which to come to terms with its body, learn to coordinate its reflexes and develop equilibrium. If it has not yet acquired biodynamic self-control, subjecting it to human requirements prematurely will inhibit neurosensory development and muscular control, impeding locomotion, and harming the normal foal's innate potential. Concentrating on specialized gestures will establish an unnatural kinetic order. The foal's acquisition of proprioception will not follow the usual spontaneous route, but be skewed towards restraint resulting in movements which are incomplete and disjointed.

The resistance that a rider may encounter from a young horse is the expression of problems arising from previous poor and non-communicating relationships. The immature foal cannot develop virtuosity if it retains painful memories. The neglect of preparatory exercise can be seen clearly in the condition of the young horse following competition. The trainer must remember the time and place when his pupil first communicates – using a recognizable signal – its awareness that it has competed well and is suffering no discomfort. To use a computing analogy, the horse must be allowed to develop its own circuits and programmes.

When a horse participating in an obstacle jumping competition enters the arena, it should set off at a leisurely and calm canter, although it is frequently not allowed to do so. The execution of a high quality jump requires excellent preparatory training, although sometimes a horse's excitement can offset biomechanical problems resulting from poor preparation.

The neurophysiological principles which govern sporting performance are identical for both man and horse. The states of proprioception and tonus, which are closely linked, reveal themselves in both good and bad movement. The execution of movement does not simply proceed from 'I want and I shall have', but from respect for all the neurophysiological aspects of performance. It has been said that 'movement is the aim of the art of equestrianism, which resides in the creation, comprehension, maintenance and guidance of the horse's efforts in a state of physical and emotional harmony'.

2 Anatomy and Basic Biomechanical Concepts

Diagnosing the symptoms of locomotor problems and devising the appropriate therapy and exercises to treat them cannot be undertaken without a deep and detailed knowledge of the anatomy and physiology of the various structures involved in locomotion, and an understanding of the way in which they work together. This combination of what could be termed the analytical and global approaches is important. Looking at the way in which the muscular and skeletal systems work together, for example, we can see how groups of muscles form chains between skeletal 'relays' which are vital to the execution of certain movements and exercises (see pages 57–61), and how composite 'ridges' formed of bone, muscle and ligament helps provide resistance against the forces generated by locomotion (see page 63). Most importantly, attention should be paid to group synergy, the way in which muscular groups which often act against each other can work together. This can be seen in the way in which flexors and extensors lock the joints in the legs when the horse lands following a jump.

This chapter is designed to provide the reader with an introduction to the the anatomic and biomechanical knowledge required to diagnose locomotor problems which benefit from physiotherapeutic treatment. Diagrams of the major anatomical regions, which also illustrate the ways in which they work together, accompany the text.

1. VERTEBRAL COLUMN

1.1 CONSTITUENT PARTS

In the horse the vertebral column consists of 7 cervical vertebrae (cervical spine, C1 - 7), 18 thoracic vertebrae (thoracic spine, T1 - 18), 6 lumbar vertebrae (lumbar spine, L1 - 6), 5 sacral vertebrae (S1 - 5) and between 18 and 22 caudal vertebrae (Fig. 6).

1. The cervical vertebrae are voluminous and long; the mobility of the neck is assisted by the hemispherical shape of the head of the vertebrae and the depth of the fossa.
2. The thoracic vertebrae have very tall spinous processes, particularly in the area around the withers where they can be 30 cm or longer; this height gives them powerful leverage. The initial orientation of these processes is dorso-caudal, becoming less pronounced at the anticlinal vertebra between T13 and T16 before changing to dorso-cranial in the lumbar area.
3. The lumbar vertebrae have very long transverse processes and their articular processes are closely interlocked, particularly in the area of L5, L6 and S1 where the processes are in contact with the synovial joints; this strongly limits lumbar mobility, particularly lateral flexion and rotation. While the orientation of the spinous process of L6 is most often dorso-

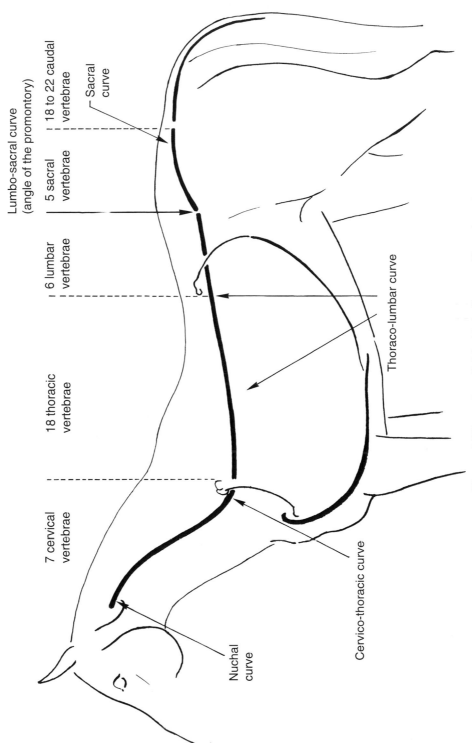

Figure 6 The spine divided into its constituent parts.

cranial, which assists lumbo-sacral mobility in flexion and extension, in many horses it is vertical, or even caudal.
4. The sacrum, which consists of the 5 sacral vertebrae fused together, is closely interconnected with both ilium bones by the powerful sacro-iliac ligaments.

(a) Spinal curves
Seen as a single unit, the vertebral column presents itself as a series of curves, the accentuation of which varies from individual to individual:

1. The nuchal (upper cervical) curve, which is dorsally convex and extends from the occipital bone to C3.
2. The cervico-thoracic (lower cervical) curve, which is ventrally convex and extends from C4 to T4.
3. The thoraco-lumbar curve (or bridge), which is usually straight if slightly dorsally convex; with saddled horses its orientation is inverted and becomes ventrally convex.
4. The lumbo-sacral curve, which is pronounced but limited to the intervertebral space between the lumbar and sacral vertebrae. The axis of the sacrum forms an angle of between 15 and 25 degrees with that of the lumbar region. This gap is visible on the horse's back as a promontory.
5. The sacral curve, dorsally convex and quite pronounced, is of little physiotherapeutic interest.

1.2 JOINTS OF THE VERTEBRAL COLUMN

(a) Intervertebral joint
An example of an intervertebral joint can be seen in Fig. 7. The interlinked bodies and arches of the vertebrae are connected to each other by powerful muscular and ligamentary attachments.

1. FUSION OF THE VERTEBRAL BODIES
This involves three principal features – the intervertebral disc, the ventral longitudinal ligament and the dorsal longitudinal ligament.

1. The intervertebral disc is narrow except in the cervical region and in the lumbar-sacral space. The fibres which constitute the Annulus fibrosus (outer fibrous ring) are attached to the apposing articular surfaces and hold them together with great force. The fibres of the central nucleus pulposus are more fibro-elastic in the horse than in other species and therefore only slightly less strong than those of the Annulus fibrosus.
2. The ventral (anterior) longitudinal ligament, absent from the atlas (the first cervical vertebra) to T5, is powerful in the thoracic, lumbar and caudal regions. It is attached to the ventral crest which projects from the lumbar vertebrae.
3. The dorsal (posterior) longitudinal ligament is thin and of little functional value.

2. FUSION OF THE VERTEBRAL ARCHES
This is achieved by synovial joints (diarthroses) between the articular processes and by ligaments.

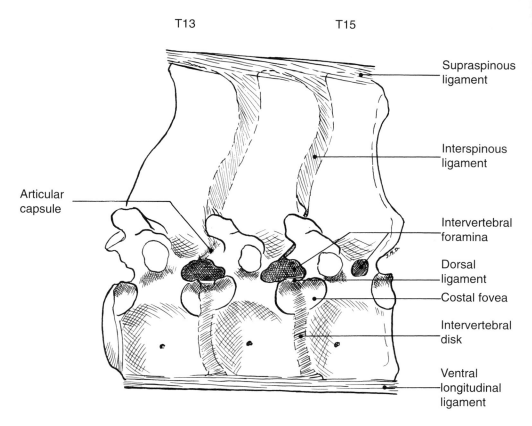

Figure 7 Example of an intervertebral joint (T13 to T15).

1. The synovial joints vary according to region. In relation to the vertebral axis the cartilaginous facets radiate outwards in the cervical region and obliquely in the thoracic region. In the lumbar region they act as sheaths, considerably limiting the possibilities for rotation and lateral flexion. The slender joint capsule is continuous with the interlamellar ligament which blocks off the entrance to the vertebral canal.
2. The interspinous ligament is short but its fibres are obliquely oriented so as not to hinder flexion and extension.
3. The supraspinous ligament is strong and its attachment to the top of the spinous processes is powerful. Its elasticity is limited in the lumbar region, but becomes pronounced in the thoracic and cervical regions, where it is continuous with the nuchal ligament.

3. MUSCULAR SUPPORT
Vertebral stability and solidity are reinforced by groups of muscles which have re-educative as well as functional capacities.

1. Closer to the spine are the juxtavertebral muscles – multifidus and intertransverse – whose rich proprioceptive innervation assists in permanent vertebral re-adjustment.

2. Further away from the spine are the epaxial and hypaxial muscles, which are usually considered antagonistic in the physiotherapeutic schema, but which work synergistically on the vertebral column when the horse is both static and active. In the cervical region they are represented by the dorsal and ventral muscles. In the lumbar region this role is played partly by the erector spinae muscle and partly by the iliopsoas muscles and those of the wall of the abdomen.

(b) Nuchal ligament

This powerful and moderately elastic ligament plays an important role in the functioning of the vertebral column. It consists of two parts (see Fig. 8):

1. The cord, which extends from the external occipital protuberance to the top of the spinous processes of the withers. After this point it is continuous with the supraspinous ligament and becomes increasingly fibrous.
2. The thick lamella, the major part of which extends from C2, C3 and C4 cranially to the spinous processes of T2, T3 and T4 caudally.

The two parts work passively yet effectively together to provide support for the head and neck, thanks to the leverage provided by the height of the thoracic spinous processes. When the head and neck are lowered, they exert a forward traction on these long lever arms causing flexion of the thoracic vertebrae (see Fig. 9).

1.3 MUSCLES OF THE NECK AND TRUNK

Two major systems which differ in both location and function can be distinguished in the muscles involved in the movement of the vertebral column:

1. The deep juxtavertebral muscles, responsible for maintaining control over the intervertebral joints, which also play a cybernetic role. With their rich proprioceptive innervation, they are the source of postural information, and thus assist in the positioning of the column. They also help regulate muscle tonus.
2. The superficial paravertebral muscles, which are less richly innervated and thus provide less information on tonus and posture. They are involved in moving joints and skeletal muscles and are appropriate for intense gymnastic effort.

(a) Muscles of the neck (Figs. 10 to 14)

The various groups of muscles in the neck can be distinguished by location and function:

1. The cervical ventral muscles, which are chiefly flexors of the neck.
2. The cervical dorsal muscles, which are principally extensors of the neck.
3. The deep juxtavertebral muscles which are involved in rotation and lateral flexion.
4. The muscles in the poll which are involved in extension and lateral flexion of the head.

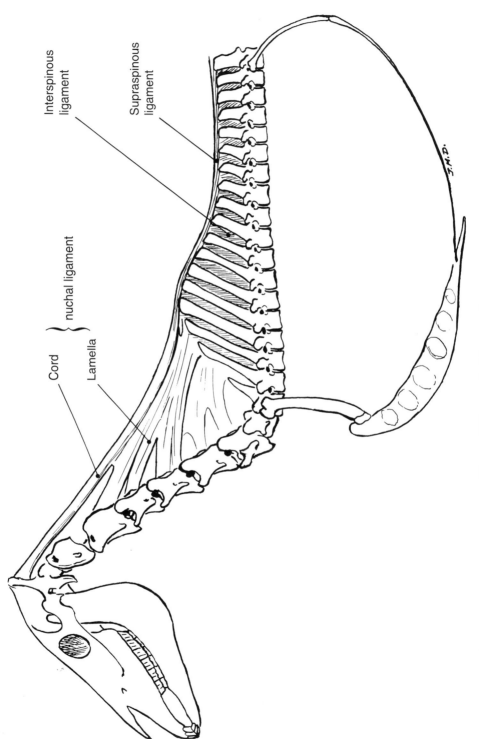

Interspinous ligament

Supraspinous ligament

Cord

} nuchal ligament

Lamella

Figure 8 The nuchal ligament.

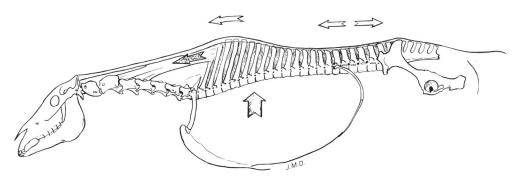

(a) Lowering the neck places the ligaments under tension, separates the thoracic spinous processes and flexes the thoracic spine.

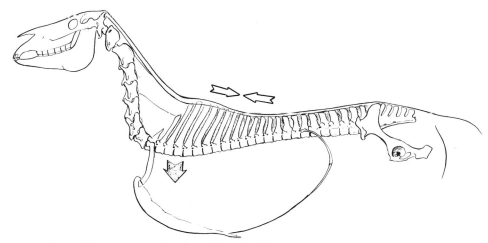

(b) Raising the neck causes cervico-thoracic extension, relaxes the ligaments, brings the spinous processes back together and extends the thoracic spine.

Figure 9 Biomechanical functioning of the nuchal and supraspinous ligaments.

1. FLEXOR MUSCLES

Brachiocephalic
ORIGIN: humeral crest.
INSERTION: mastoid process of the temporal bone.
ACTION: fixed point at insertion – protraction of the forelimb, control of the extent of the gait, initiator of rearward movement; fixed point at origin – contracted bilaterally, flexion of the neck and extension of the poll; contracted unilaterally, lateral flexion and rotation of the neck and poll.

Sternocephalic
ORIGIN: sternal manubrium.
INSERTION: caudal rim of the ramus of the mandible.
ACTION: contracted bilaterally, flexion of neck and poll; contracted unilaterally, lateral flexion and rotation of the neck and head.

Scalenus
ORIGIN: first rib.
INSERTION: transverse processes of last four cervical vertebrae.
ACTION: fixed point at insertion – respiration (inspiration); fixed point at origin – contracted bilaterally, flexion of the base of the neck (C4 to T1); contracted unilaterally, lateral flexion and rotation of the same region.

Longus capitis (long muscle of the head)
ORIGIN: transverse processes of C3 to C5.
INSERTION: tubercle of the occipital bone.
ACTION: contracted bilaterally, flexion of the poll; contracted unilaterally, rotation and lateral flexion of the upper cervical vertebrae.

2. EXTENSOR MUSCLES

Trapezius
ORIGIN: nuchal cord and supraspinous ligament.
INSERTION: spine of the scapula.
ACTION: fixed point at insertion – minor contribution to the extension and lateral movements of the neck; fixed point at origin – major contribution to movements of the dorsal extremity of the scapula at the various gaits.

Omotransverse
ORIGIN: spine of the scapula and the humeral crest.
INSERTION: cervical transverse processes.
ACTION: fixed point at origin – contracted bilaterally, slight extension of the neck; contracted unilaterally, lateral flexion of the neck; fixed point at insertion – protraction of the forelimb (together with the brachiocephalic).

Rhomboid
ORIGIN: nuchal cord and the top of the spinous processes of the first thoracic vertebrae.
INSERTION: medial side of the cartilage of the scapula.
ACTION: fixed point at origin – drawing the scapula forward; fixed point at insertion – contracted bilaterally, contributes to the extension of the lower cervical area; contracted unilaterally, lateral movements of the neck.

Cervical serratus
ORIGIN: tranverse processes of C3 to C7.
INSERTION: serrated cranial surface of the scapula.
ACTION: fixed point at origin – cranially and ventrally drawing the dorsal extremity of the scapula towards the neck; fixed point at insertion – contracted bilaterally, supports the base of the neck, extensor of the lower cervical region; contracted unilaterally, rotates the lower cervical vertebrae.

Splenius
ORIGIN: thoraco-lumbar fascia; top of spinous processes from T3 to T5.
INSERTION: mastoidal crest, caudal tubercle of the wing of atlas and transverse processes of C2 to C5.
ACTION: fixed point at insertion – contracted bilaterally, elevation of the head, extension of the poll and neck; contracted unilaterally, rotation and lateral flexion of the cervical vertebrae.

Semispinalis capitis (large complexus)
ORIGIN: thoraco-lumbar fascia, top of the first thoracic spinous processes, transverse processes from T3 to T7, articular processes from C2 to C7.
INSERTION: external occipital protuberance.
ACTION: fixed point at insertion – tensor of the thoraco-lumbar fascia, raising of the base of the neck; fixed point at origin – contracted bilaterally, powerful extensor of the poll and neck; contracted unilaterally, rotation and lateral flexion of the cervical vertebrae.

Longissimus capitis and atlantis (small complexus)
ORIGIN: transverse processes of T1 and T2; articular processes from C2 to C7.
INSERTION: mastoidal process; caudal tubercle of the wing of the atlas.
ACTION: contracted bilaterally, extensor of the poll and neck; contracted unilaterally, lateral flexion and rotation of the poll and neck.

Spinalis cervicis
ORIGIN: spinous processes of T1 to T3.
INSERTION: spinous processes of C4 to C7.
ACTION: extensor of the cervico-thoracic region.

3. JUXTAVERTEBRAL MUSCLES
While these are less important for physiotherapeutic purposes, due to their smaller size and less powerful attachments, they play an important role in the maintenance of intervertebral stability. They are also richly innervated and thus key cybernetic muscles, involved in proprioception while the horse is both static and active.

Longus colli (long muscle of the neck)
INSERTIONS: vertebral bodies from the axis to C7 and T1 to T6; terminal tendon on the ventral tubercle of the atlas.
ACTION: flexion and rotation of the cervical and cranial thoracic vertebrae.

Multifidus cervicis
ORIGIN: transverse processes of the cervical vertebrae.
INSERTION: spinous processes of the cervical vertebrae.
ACTION: stabilizing of joints; rotation and cervical lateral flexion; weak extensor action.

Intertransverse
INSERTIONS: stretched between the transverse processes of adjacent vertebrae.
ACTION: lateral flexion and cervical rotation.

4. MUSCLES OF THE POLL

Dorsal straight muscles (major and minor) of the head
ORIGIN: spinous processes of the axis (major) and dorsal arch of the atlas (minor).
INSERTION: external occipital protuberance.
ACTION: extensor of the poll.

Caudal oblique muscle of the head
ORIGIN: side of the spinous process of the axis.
INSERTION: dorsal side of the wing of the atlas.
ACTION: contracted unilaterally, rotation and atlanto-axial lateral flexion; contracted bilaterally, atlanto-axial extension.

Lateral and ventral straight muscles of the head
Situated ventrally to the atlanto-occipital joint, these are involved in the flexion of the head.

(b) Muscles of the trunk

In this vast area, as in the neck, it is important to identify the various muscular groups. The deep, cybernetic juxtavertebral muscles are involved in proprioception. Their state of tension or stretching modulates the activity of the much more powerful superficial muscle groups, which have a greater determining impact on posture and movement. Some of the muscles which are ventral to the vertebral column are flexors of the thoraco-lumbar bridge; those which are dorsal are extensors of the same area. All are involved to a greater or lesser extent in lateral flexion and rotation.

1. FLEXOR MUSCLES

Two groups of muscles can be distinguished, in the wall of the abdomen and in the lumbo-iliac region.

1.1 Muscles in the wall of the abdomen

These hold the abdominal viscera in place and are involved in respiration (expiration). As they are not very thick their impact on locomotion is due to their length and the fact that their extensions are eccentric in relation to the vertebral axis; they are thus able to act on other more powerful muscles.

External oblique (obliquus externus)
ORIGIN: lateral side of the ribs (6th to 18th).
INSERTION: linea alba; inguinal archway.
ACTION: contracted bilaterally, flexion of the thoraco-lumbar spine; contracted unilaterally, lateral flexion (curving inwards) and rotation.

Internal oblique (obliquus internus)
ORIGIN: ventro-cranial iliac spine (angle of the hip) and inguinal archway.
INSERTION: medial side of the distal extremity of the last four or five ribs.
ACTION: working together with the oblique external muscle on the same side to produce flexion and lateral flexion of the vertebral column; working against this muscle during thoraco-lumbar rotation.

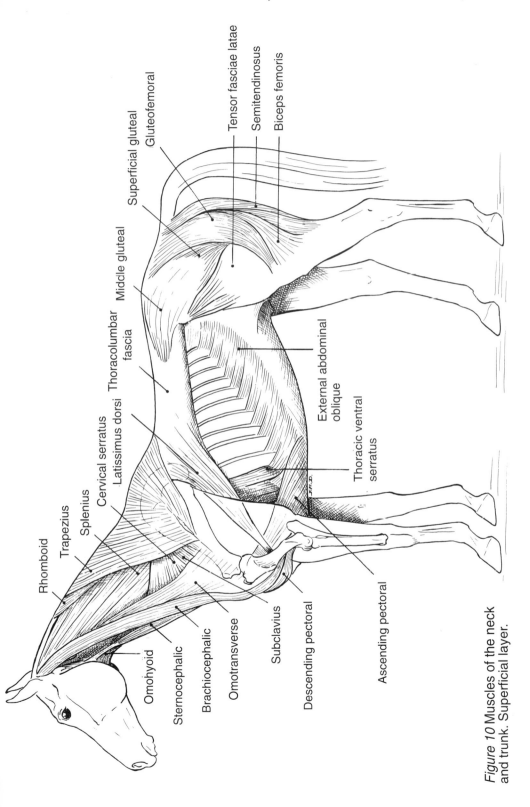

Figure 10 Muscles of the neck and trunk. Superficial layer.

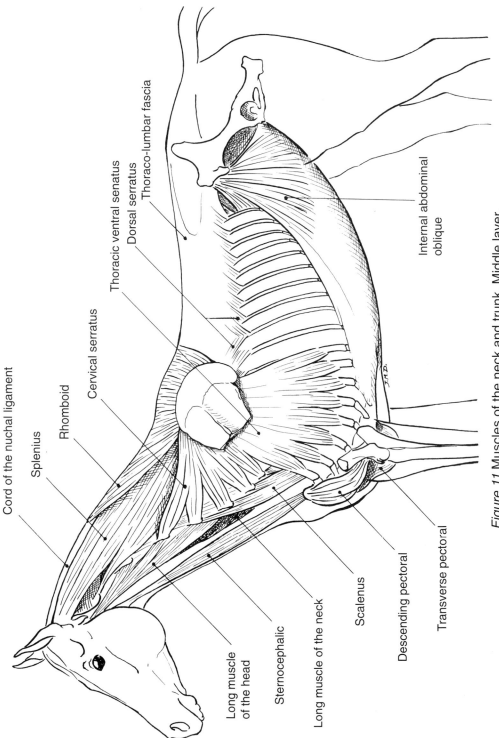

Cord of the nuchal ligament

Splenius

Rhomboid

Cervical serratus

Thoracic ventral senatus

Dorsal serratus

Thoraco-lumbar fascia

Internal abdominal oblique

Long muscle of the head

Sternocephalic

Long muscle of the neck

Scalenus

Descending pectoral

Transverse pectoral

Figure 11 Muscles of the neck and trunk. Middle layer.

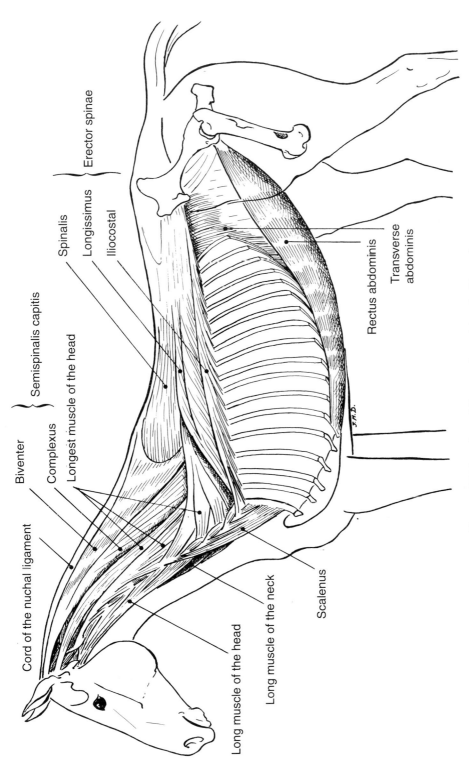

Cord of the nuchal ligament

Biventer
Complexus
Longest muscle of the head

Semispinalis capitis

Spinalis
Longissimus
Iliocostal

Erector spinae

Long muscle of the head

Long muscle of the neck

Scalenus

Rectus abdominis

Transverse
abdominis

Figure 12 Muscles of the neck and trunk. Deep layer.

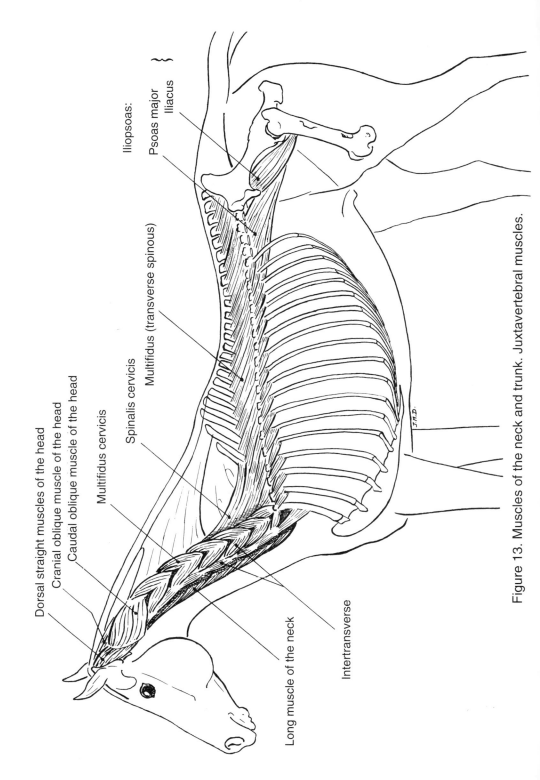

Figure 13. Muscles of the neck and trunk. Juxtavertebral muscles.

Iliopsoas:
Psoas major
Iliacus

Multifidus (transverse spinous)

Spinalis cervicis

Multifidus cervicis

Dorsal straight muscles of the head
Cranial oblique muscle of the head
Caudal oblique muscle of the head

Long muscle of the neck

Intertransverse

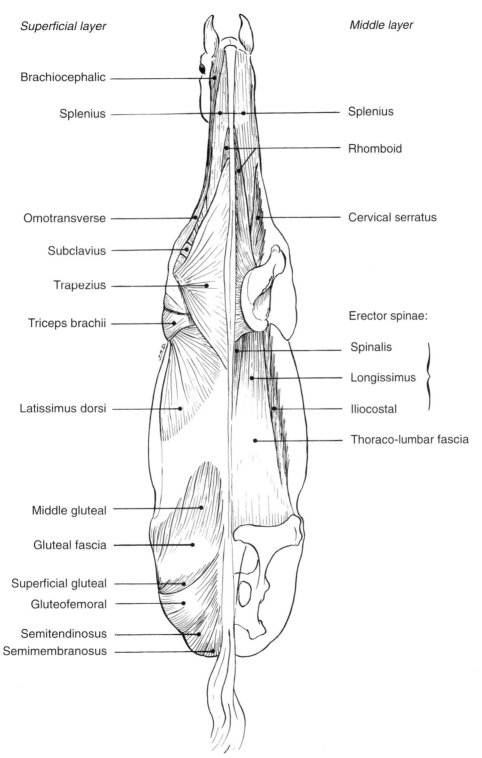

Superficial layer

Brachiocephalic

Splenius

Omotransverse

Subclavius

Trapezius

Triceps brachii

Latissimus dorsi

Middle gluteal

Gluteal fascia

Superficial gluteal
Gluteofemoral

Semitendinosus
Semimembranosus

Middle layer

Splenius

Rhomboid

Cervical serratus

Erector spinae:

Spinalis

Longissimus

Iliocostal

Thoraco-lumbar fascia

ﬁgure 14 Muscles of the neck and trunk. Dorsal view.

Rectus abdominis
ORIGIN: sternum; costal cartilages of ribs 4 to 9.
INSERTION: cranial rim of the pubis and the prepubic tendon.
ACTION: flexion of the thoraco-lumbar-sacral sections of the column; contracted unilaterally, slight bending and rotation of the same area.

Transverse abdominis
ORIGIN: transverse processes of the lumbar vertebrae and costal cartilages.
INSERTION: linea alba.
ACTION: working together with all the preceding muscles, assisting the abdominal cavity in its role as a support for the proper functioning of the vertebral column.

1.2 Muscles of the lumbo-iliac region
Note: as it is not involved in the movement of the spinal column, the iliac muscle is not discussed in this chapter.

Psoas major
ORIGIN: ventral side of the transverse processes of the lumbar vertebrae and the last two ribs.
INSERTION: minor trochanter of the femur.
ACTION: flexion of the lumbo-sacral joint, the lumbar spine and the sacro-iliac joint; contracted unilaterally, rotation and lateral flexion of the lumbar spine; coxo-femoral (hip) flexion and lateral rotation of the femur.

Psoas minor
ORIGIN: ventral side of the vetebral bodies from T16 to L5.
INSERTION: tuberosity on the cervix of the ilium.
ACTION: flexion of the lumbo-sacral and sacro-iliac joints.

Quadratus lumborum
ORIGIN: iliac crest.
INSERTION: ventral side of the lumbar transverse processes.
ACTION: lateral flexion of the lumbar region.

2. EXTENSOR MUSCLES
These three muscles, collectively known as erector spinae, are contained within the thoraco-lumbar fascia, itself placed under tension by the cranial and caudal scrratus muscles in the thorax. This powerful muscular mass originates at the iliac crest, the dorsal side of the thoracic and lumbar transverse processes and at the dorsal extremity of the ribs. The group divides at the cranial end into the three muscles, which are distinguished by their location, points of insertion and action.

Iliocostal
SITUATION: on the outside of the group.
INSERTION: tuberosities in 18 ribs, and the last cervical transverse process.
ACTION: primarily expiration and thoraco-lumbar lateral flexion.

Longissimus dorsi
SITUATION: between the other two muscles.
INSERTION: thoracic and lumbar transverse processes; dorsal extremity of the ribs.
ACTION: vertebral extension and lateral flexion.

Spinalis thoracis
SITUATION: on the inside of the group.
INSERTION: thoracic spinous processes.
ACTION: extension of the thoraco-lumbar spine.

3. JUXTAVERTEBRAL MUSCLES

Multifidus (transverse spinous)
This muscle is formed of multiple bundles that overlap each other obliquely.
ORIGIN: thoracic and lumbar transverse processes.
INSERTION: spinous processes of the 2 or 3 vertebrae preceding the origin.
ACTION: support of the joints and proprioception; lateral flexion and rotation of the intervertebral spaces; weak extensor action.

1.4 VERTEBRAL BIOMECHANICS

Biomechanical interactions between the cervical spine and the thoraco-lumbar bridge have already been mentioned (see Fig. 9). These two major regions are now looked at in greater detail.

(a) Cervical spine

The amplitude of the movements of the intervertebral joints in the neck is clearly greater than that of the thoraco-lumbar bridge. This functional difference is due principally to the following factors:

1. The structure of the vertebral heads and fossae, which are quasi-hemispherical in this area.
2. The greater thickness of the intervertebral discs.
3. The flattened shape of the surfaces of the dorsal articular processes.
4. The lower crests of the spinous processes.
5. The elasticity of the nuchal ligament, which is superior to that of the interspinous and supraspinous ligaments.
6. The absence of the ventral longitudinal ligament, the function of which is taken over by longus colli.

At either end of the cervical section are features which enhance the mobility of its central part. The atlanto-occipital and atlanto-axial joints, with their specialized movements, and the differentiation of specific muscles (caudal and oblique straight muscles of the head) provide the nuchal region with the ability to move the head in any direction. The thickness of the intervertebral discs and the shape of the articular surfaces equip the thoraco-cervical junction between C5 and T2 with its great capacity to maintain control of the cervico-cephalic region.

1. FLEXION AND EXTENSION

1.1 Physiology

Flexion and extension are given greater scope in the area around the atlanto-occipital joint and in the intervertebral spaces between C5 and T1.

1. During *flexion*, a vertebral fossa slides ventrally against the head of its neighbour (Fig. 15), causing the latter to jut into the intervertebral canal which becomes narrower as a result. The intervertebral disc is subjected to shearing pressures. The height of the intervertebral foramina is increased by the sliding action, the overlap between dorsal joint facets is reduced and the joint capsule is placed under tension. The nuchal ligament is stretched.
2. During *extension*, all these mechanical phenomena are reversed. The head of a vertebra slides ventrally against the fossa of the preceding vertebra. The intervertebral canal increases in size. The shearing pressures on the disc operate in the opposite direction. The height of the intervertebral foramina diminishes, reducing the space available to the large cervical nerve fibres passing through them. The overlap between dorsal joint facets is increased and the nuchal ligament is relaxed.

1.2 Muscles involved

1. The flexor muscles are illustrated in Fig. 16. Flexion of the cervico-thoracic area is caused by the bilateral action of the scalenus, long muscle of the neck and sternocephalic muscles. The brachiocephalic muscle is also involved, although its primary function is to move the forelimb. Flexion of the upper cervical area is principally effected by concentric contraction of the long muscles of the head and neck and sternocephalic muscles.
2. The extensor muscles are illustrated in Fig. 17. Extension of the cervico-thoracic area (raising of the neck) is the product of joint bilateral concentric contraction (with insertion as the fixed point), of the erector spinae and cervical dorsal muscles. Extension of the upper cervical area is effected by the splenius and semispinalis muscles, as well as by the dorsal and oblique straight muscles of the head.

2. LATERAL FLEXION AND ROTATION

2.1 Physiology

With the intervertebral joints, as with the majority of the joints in the horse, these two actions are connected. As with flexion and extension, the amplitude of movement is greater in the lower cervical and nuchal areas. With the exception of the nuchal area any lateral flexion (i.e. curving inwards) is accompanied by rotation of the vertebral bodies in the *opposite* direction. The direction of rotation is determined by the side towards which the ventral crest of a vertebral body moves in relation to the neighbouring vertebra if the latter is treated as a fixed point. In the nuchal area, rotation is largely effected via the atlanto-axial joint and lateral flexion via the atlanto-occipital joint. In fact, these movements cannot be separated mechanically, and lateral flexion of the head involves lateral rotation of the atlas in relation to the axis and contralateral rotation of the occipital in relation to the atlas (Fig. 18). The atlas can be thought of as a buffer placed between the cranial extremity of the vertebral column and the head. During lateral flexion of the neck, its lateral rotation compensates for the contralateral rotation of the rest of the cervical column and allows the head to remain facing the same direction.

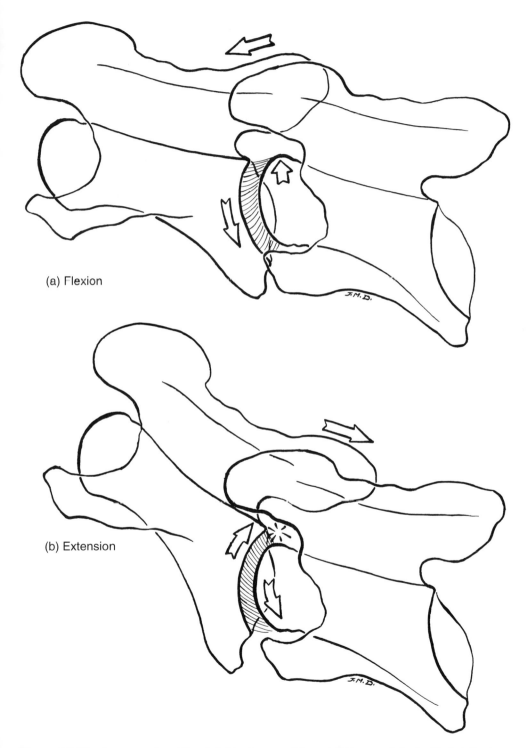

Figure 15 Displacements of the joint between C5 and C6 associated with (a) flexion and (b) extension (adapted from radiographs).

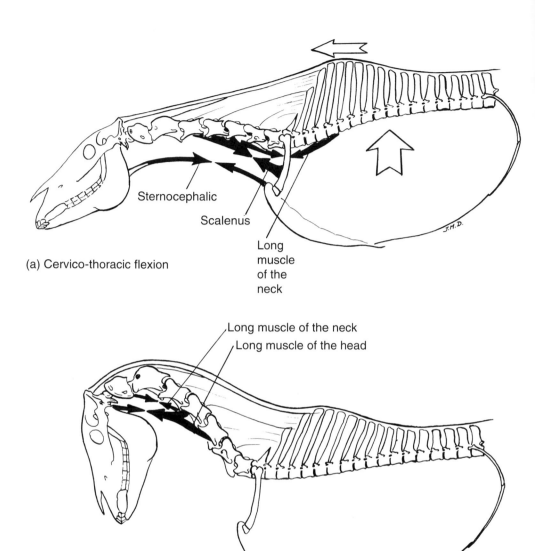

Sternocephalic

Scalenus

Long
muscle
of the
neck

(a) Cervico-thoracic flexion

Long muscle of the neck
Long muscle of the head

(b) Upper cervical area flexion

Figure 16 Muscles involved in flexing the neck. Flexion of the (a) cervico-thoracic
and (b) upper cervical areas.

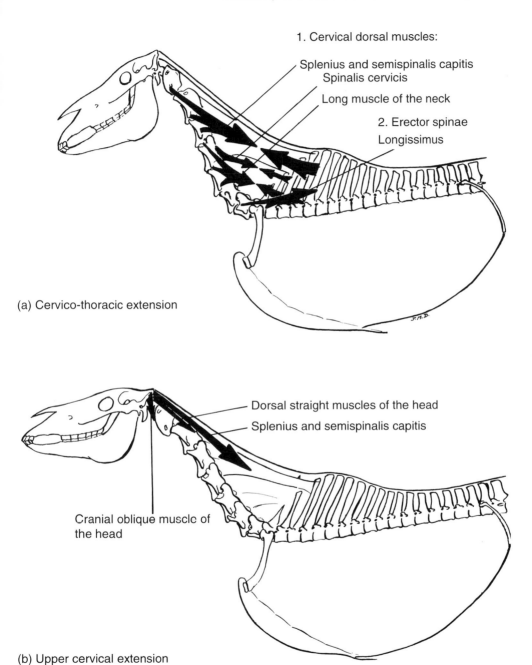

1. Cervical dorsal muscles:

Splenius and semispinalis capitis
Spinalis cervicis

Long muscle of the neck

2. Erector spinae

Longissimus

(a) Cervico-thoracic extension

Dorsal straight muscles of the head

Splenius and semispinalis capitis

Cranial oblique muscle of the head

(b) Upper cervical extension

Figure 17 Muscles involved in extending the neck. Extension of the (a) cervico-thoracic and (b) upper cervical areas.

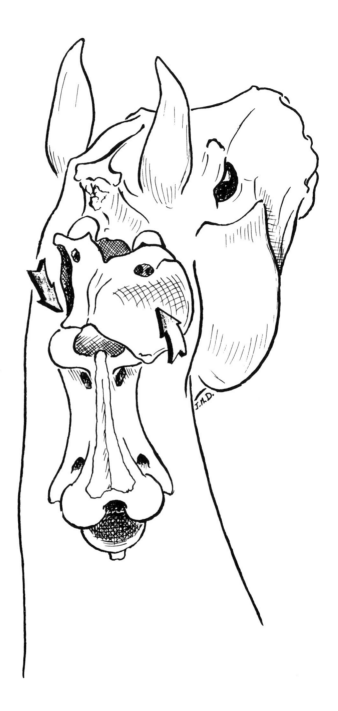

Figure 18 Movements associated with rotation and lateral flexion of the cervico-cephalic junction.

2.2 Muscles involved

Cervical *lateral flexion* (Fig. 19) is the product of joint unilateral concentric contraction of the ventral cervical muscles, such as the scalenus and sternocephalic muscles, and the majority of the dorsal cervical muscles. When the scalenus and dorsal cervical muscles are at their most extended, their insertions reveal clearly the movements of contralateral rotation; the spinous processes, in particular, contribute to the concavity of the movement. Rotation is assisted by specific muscles such as multifidus cervicis.

In the nuchal region both of these movements are produced by concentric contraction of the cranial and caudal oblique and dorsal straight muscles of the head. They are assisted by the long cervical muscles, the splenius, semispinalis and brachiocephalic.

(b) Thoraco-lumbar spine

1. PHYSIOLOGY

There are obstacles to flexibility between the cervical and thoraco-lumbar spines; assessing the global role of the thoraco-lumbar bridge should not be undertaken without first looking at the effects of positioning the neck. The mechanics of the intervertebral joints are considered below, in section 1.2.

1.1 Thoraco-lumbar bridge

Flexion and extension
The ideas presented in this section have been taken from studies which involved using freshly dissected cadavers; muscular actions were duplicated by using rubber expanders (Fig. 20).

Flexion (Fig. 21)
Exerting tension on the rectus abdominis muscle between the pubis and the sternum reveals the existence of two anatomical features which are vital to mobility in this area:

1. The *lumbo-sacral hinge joint*. Its situation varies between L5 and S1 according to individual conformation of L6 and the intervertebral spaces between L5 and L6 and L6 and S1. Mobility is enhanced by the greater elasticity of the supraspinous and interspinous ligaments, and by the thickness of the last intervertebral disc.
2. The thoraco-lumbar junction. Radiographic pictures reveal that intervertebral mobility in the column between T5 and L5 is greatest in the section between T17 and L2.

Extension (Fig. 21)
Reproducing the movement of the muscles of the erector spinae group confirms that the lumbo-sacral hinge joint offers the greatest latitude for extension; this is made possible by the way in which the spinous processes move away from each other. The thoraco-lumbar junction allows the greatest latitude for movement within the thoracic and lumbar regions.

Lowering the neck (cervico-thoracic flexion) (Fig. 22)
This action, which makes the cervical spine horizontal, automatically involves flexion of the thoracic section as well. It is the product of the traction exerted by the nuchal cord and lamella on the spinous processes of the first thoracic vertebrae. The latter simultaneously move apart and the vertebral arches bend.

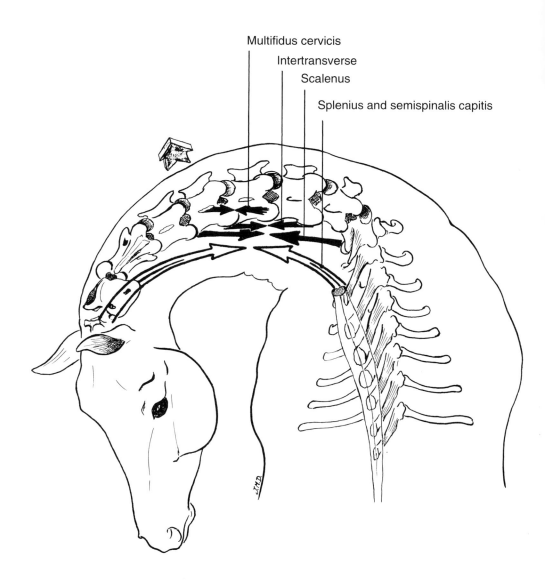

Multifidus cervicis

Intertransverse

Scalenus

Splenius and semispinalis capitis

Figure 19 Cervical lateral flexion

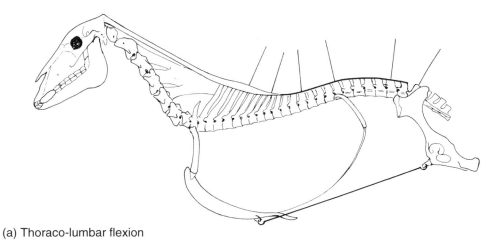

(a) Thoraco-lumbar flexion

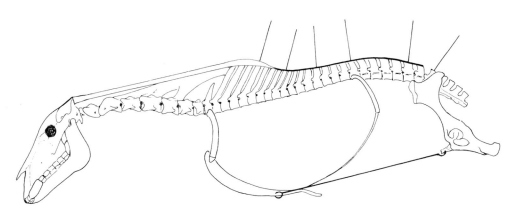

(b) Cervical and thoraco-lumbar flexion

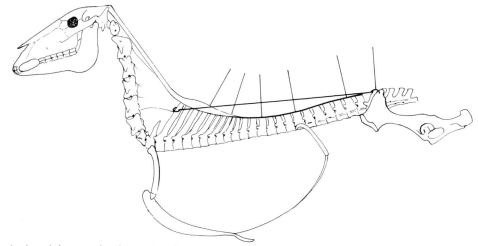

(c) Cervical and thoraco-lumbar extension

Figure 20 Reproduction, using rubber straps, of the movements of flexion and extension.

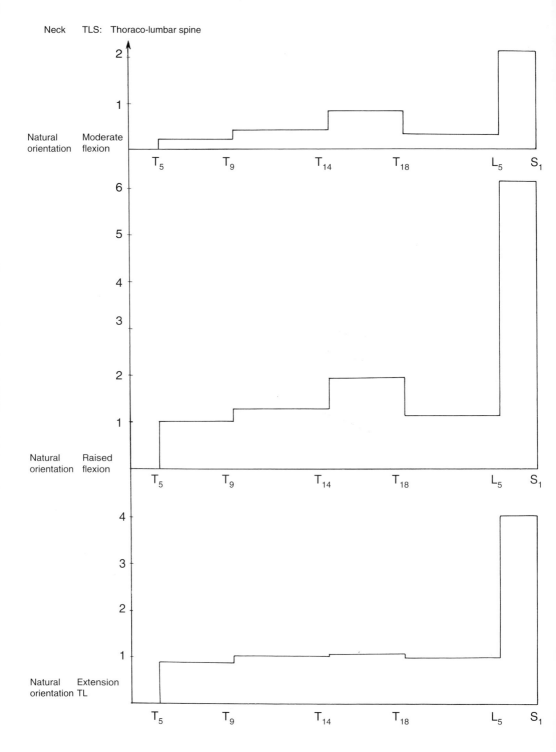

Figure 21 Mobility in the thoraco-lumbar spine. Median value of dorso-ventral movements within the intervertebral spaces in each section.

Cervical and thoraco-lumbar flexion (Figs. 20, 22)

Lowering of the neck, when accompanied by the application of tension to the sterno-pubic area, also places the supraspinous ligament under tension, revealing the relative rigidity of the lumbar area. The lumbo-sacral joint remains mobile, which is notable, given the pressure exerted by thoraco-lumbar flexion.

Movements in the thoracic region involve different sections of the spine. The thoraco-lumbar junction is not involved unless tension is being exerted in the sterno-pubic area.

The foregoing paragraphs emphasize a number of features of the vertebral biomechanics of the Horse. The principal consequences of lowering the neck are as follows:

1. Moving apart of the thoracic spinous processes.
2. Forward traction of the nuchal ligament, which places the supraspinous ligament under tension, causing the lumbar area to lock; this locking increases the work of the abdominal muscles and necessitates compensatory action by the lumbo-sacral and coxo-femoral (hip) joints.

It is worth mentioning that the minor movements of flexion and extension in the area around the sacro-iliac joint are generally associated with those of the lumbo-sacral hinge joint and are determined by the same muscular groups.

Lateral flexion and rotation

The only studies which have quantified lateral movements and rotation of the vertebral column are those of Townsend and Leach (1983). According to these authors (Fig. 23), the scope for these movements is greatest in the lower half of the thoracic spine, approximately between T9 and T14.

1.2 Mechanics of the thoraco-lumbar intervertebral joints

Investigations to date have had as their focus the identification of instantaneous centres of rotation (ICR) for all movements in the median plane (Denoix, 1986). It is worth noting that the specific ICRs involved in lateral flexion and rotation are much more difficult to identify due to the fact that these movements are always interlinked. During flexion and rotation, the ICR of a particular thoracic or lumbar vertebra – the point around which it moves in the median plane – is almost always located in the body of the following vertebra (Figs. 24, 25). This affects the nature of the associated movements of the various parts of the vertebrae and the intervertebral joints (Fig. 26).

The action of *flexion* has the following global consequences, each of which are considered in relation to the following vertebra being treated as a fixed point:

1. The vertebral body slides ventrally and the intervertebral disc is subjected to shearing forces. The ventral longitudinal ligament is relaxed but its fibres become oblique at its various points of insertion.
2. At the level of the vertebral arches, the spinous processes diverge, placing the supraspinous ligament under tension. The interspinous ligament is subject to relatively few constraints on account of the radial orientation of its fibres relative to the ICR. The dorsal synovial joints slide away from each other, according to the orientation of the articular facets and the position of the ICR.
3. Between these two levels, the intervertebral foramen, when it is not isolated by a bony relay, tends to widen.

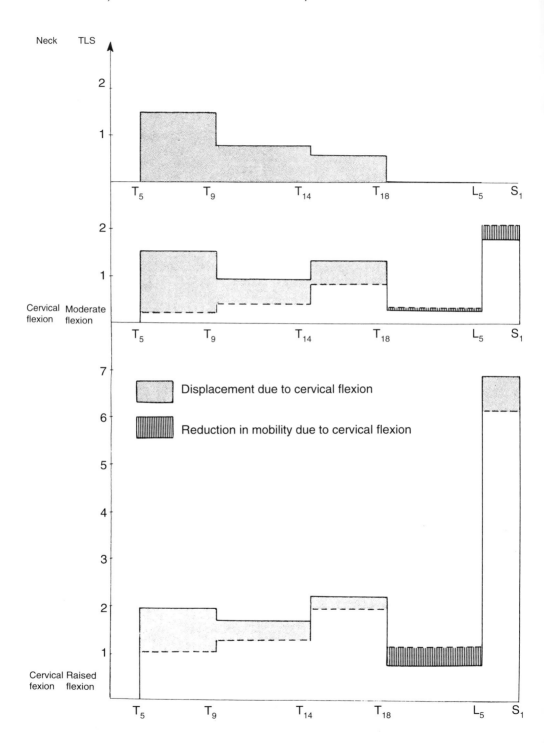

Figure 22 Mobility in the thoraco-lumbar spine when the neck is lowered. Median value of dorso-ventral movements within the intervertebral spaces in each section.

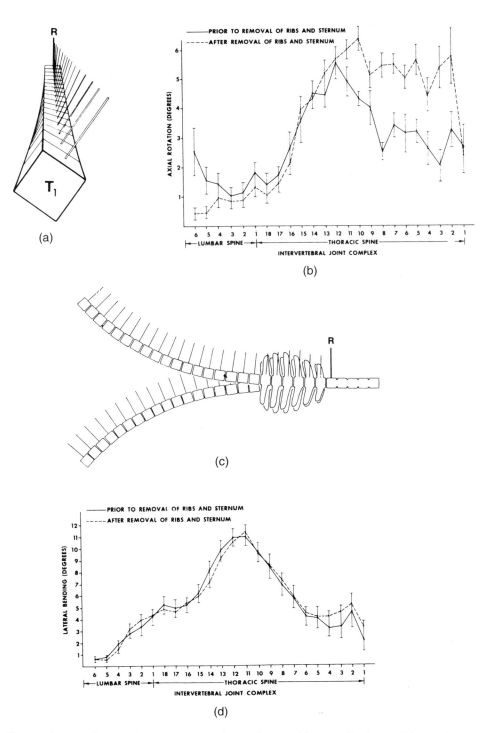

Figure 23 Amplitude of movements of rotation and lateral-flexion within each intervertebral space in the thoraco-lumbar spine (After Townsend, Leach and Fretz, 1983).

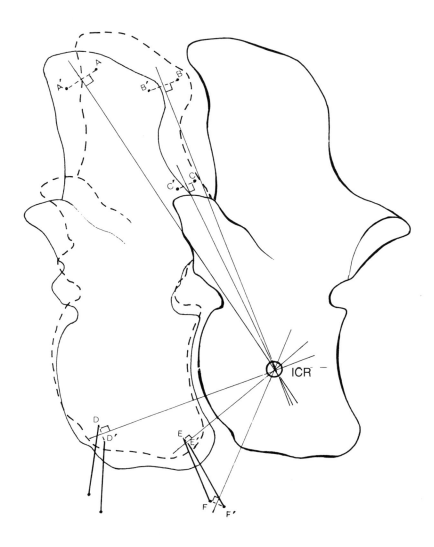

Figure 24 Diagrammatic method of determining ICR within intervertebral spaces for each dorso-ventral movement of the vertebral column.

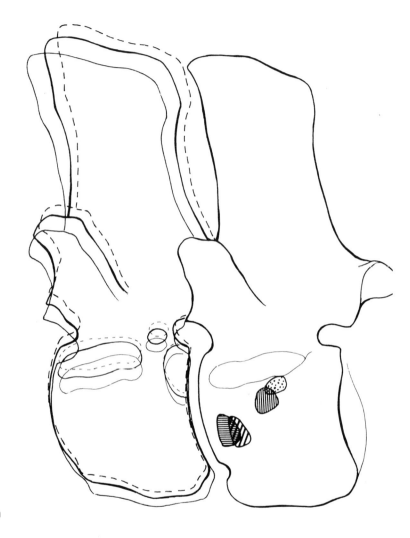

⊙ Extension

⬚ Thoraco-lumbar flexion

⊜ Cervical flexion

⬚ Cervical and throaco-lumbar flexion

Figure 25 Intervertebral space between T17 and T18. ICR of dorso-ventral movements of the vertebral column.

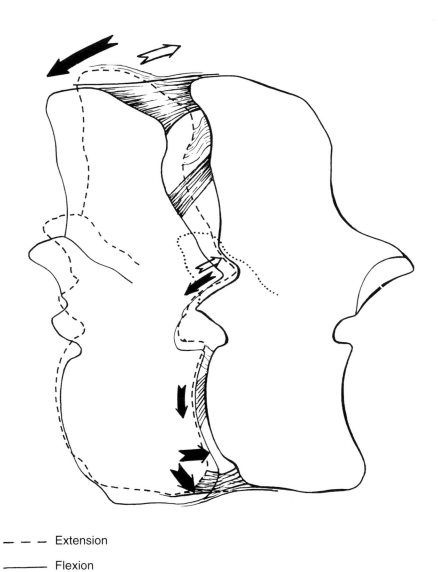

— — — Extension

———— Flexion

Figure 26 Movements within an intervertebral space during dorso-ventral flexion and rotation.

During *extension* the above movements clearly happen in reverse:

1. The body of each vertebra rises in relation to the one following, and the intervertebral disc is subjected to shearing forces which work in the opposite direction.
2. The ventral longitudinal ligament is stretched, and the supraspinous ligament is relaxed. The facets of the dorsal synovial joints move into alignment with each other.
3. The intervertebral foramen narrows.

With regard to the lumbo-sacral intervertebral space (Fig. 27), the ICR associated with flexion and extension is closer to the disc, reminiscent of the position in which it occurs in humans (Gonon *et al.*). One particular result of this is that the dorso-ventral movements of L6, in relation to S1, are less ample, and that the shearing forces operating on the disc tend to be replaced by the forces of traction and compression. The most important aspect of the thickness of this disc lies perhaps in its connection with these functional roles.

2. MUSCLES INVOLVED

2.1 Flexion (Fig. 28)
The flexor muscles of the thoraco-lumbar spine can be divided into the following groups, in terms of their location, insertion and action:

1. The muscles of the latero-ventral wall of the abdomen (rectus and internal oblique), which extend their insertions from the sternum to the pubis. Via their attachment to the ribs they are flexors of the whole section, particularly the hinge joint between T7 and L2 and the lumbo-sacral hinge joint.
2. The muscles of the lower lumbar region (psoas) extend, cranially, no further than T16 and the 17th rib; they are essentially flexors of the lumbo-sacral hinge joint.

2.2 Extension (Fig. 29)
These muscles are similarly divided according to location and function:

1. The muscles of the erector spinae group (particularly longissimus and spinalis) with their extensive insertions, and multifidus, are extensors of the whole section. Erector spinae is also an extensor of the lumbo-sacral hinge joint.
2. The hinge joint also benefits from the powerful action of the middle gluteal; this muscle, via its cranial attachments to the thoraco-lumbar fascia, is used to bring the pelvis into alignment with the vertebral axis.

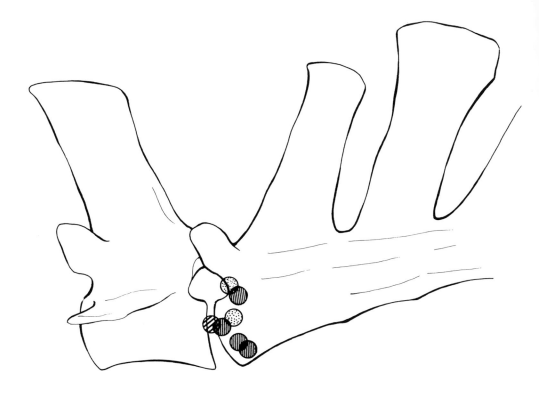

 Extension

Thoraco-lumbar flexion

Cervical and thoraco-lumbar flexion

Figure 27 Lumbo-sacral articulation. ICR of dorso-ventral movements of the
vertebral column.

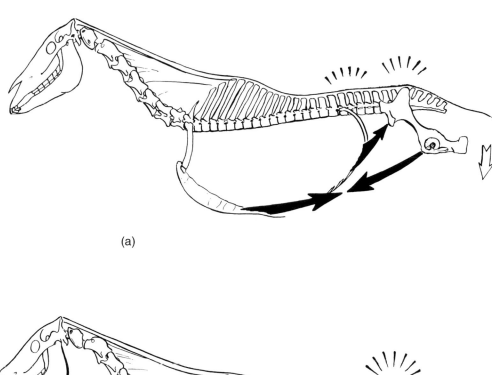

(a)

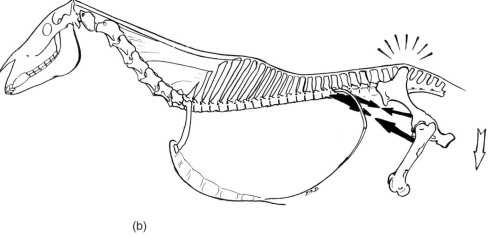

(b)

Figure 28 Flexors of the vertebral column. (a) Thoraco-lumbar and lumbo-sacral flexion; concentric contraction of the rectus and internal oblique muscles of the abdomen. (b) Lumbo-sacral flexion; concentric contraction of psoas major and minor.

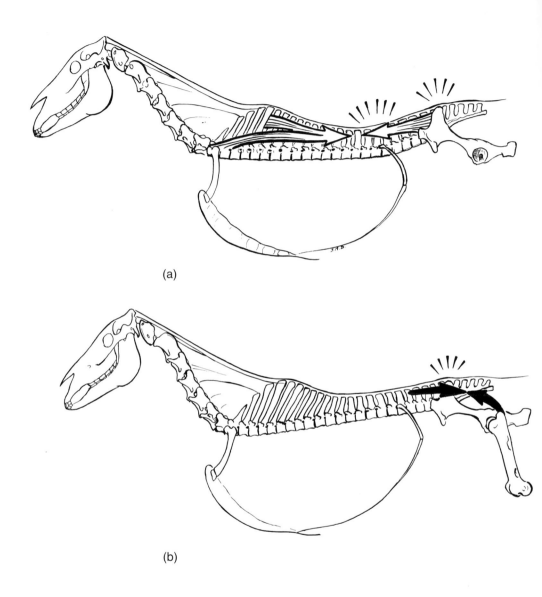

(a)

(b)

Figure 29 Muscles responsible for extension of the vertebral column. (a) Thoraco-lumbar and lumbo-sacral extension: longissimus and spinalis of the erector spinae. (b) Lumbo-sacral extension: middle gluteal.

2.3 Lateral flexion (Fig. 30)

This movement is essentially produced by the iliocostal and longissimus muscles of the erector spinae group and by the oblique abdominal muscles. The psoas and quadratus muscles of the loins contribute in only a minor capacity, as the possibility of inward curvation in the lumbar region is minimal.

2.4 Rotation (Fig. 31)

The movements involved in rotation and lateral flexion are always linked, and all the muscles mentioned above are also rotators of the vertebral column.

The muscles most adapted to inducing thoraco-lumbar torsion are multifidus and the oblique abdominals. It is, therefore, worth noting that the oblique muscles on the same side work *synergistically* during lateral flexion, but *antagonistically* during rotation. During the latter the internal oblique of one side moves in the same direction as the external oblique and contralateral multifidus muscles.

1.5 SYNTHESIS

(a) The concept of muscular chains (Fig. 32)

Muscular traction leaves a series of imprints on the skeleton, in which anchorage points develop. The vertebral spinous and transverse processes illustrate this process well. These levers serve as relays for muscular chains which extend dorsally and ventrally along the vertebral axis.

1. DORSAL CHAIN

1.1 Constituent parts

1. Cervical dorsal muscles involved in lifting the neck and which are extensors of the cervico-thoracic hinge joint.
2. The erector spinae and multifidus muscles, which are extensors of the thoraco-lumbar spine.
3. The gluteal and caudal femoral muscles, which are extensors of the hip.

1.2 Anchorage points

This powerful vertebral muscular chain converges on the three high spinous processes at the withers which act as a solid point of anchorage for the cervico-thoracic hinge joint. Caudally, there is a second, pelvic, anchorage point, which is formed by the pelvic bones and which makes possible the establishment of continuity between the vertebral and ischio-tibial (or caudal femoral) muscular chains, the attachments of which extend as far as the insertions of the caudal femoral muscles.

1.3 Action

This continuity plays a commanding role in the numerous movements involved in impulsion, jumping and leaping. During these exercises, the different parts of the chain work together. From the area of the stifle, they pull on the pelvis, and from the pelvis they pull on the cervico-thoracic anchorage point to lift the forclimb.

With regard to the horse's behaviour, tenseness in this muscular grouping is indicative of alertness or anxiety. Psychological problems, conflict, resistance to commands and disobedience are manifested here. It is also the grouping which provides evidence of the horse

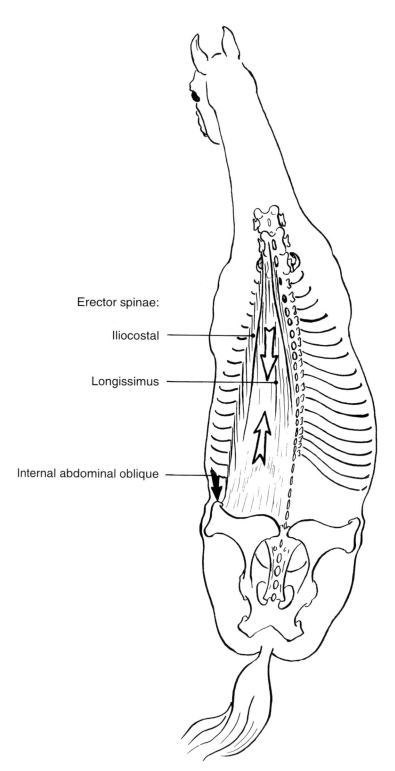

Erector spinae:

Iliocostal

Longissimus

Internal abdominal oblique

Figure 30 Muscles responsible for vertebral lateral flexion.

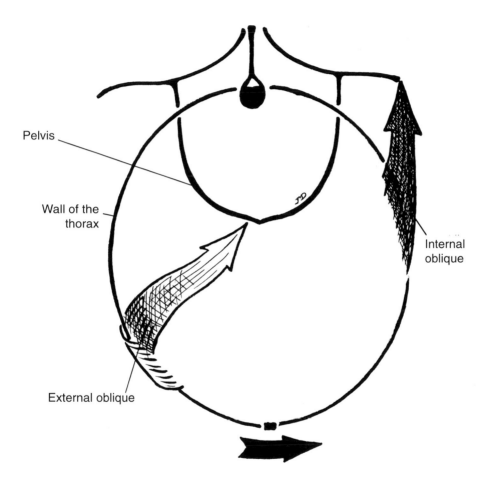

Figure 31 Rotatory function of the oblique abdominal muscles.

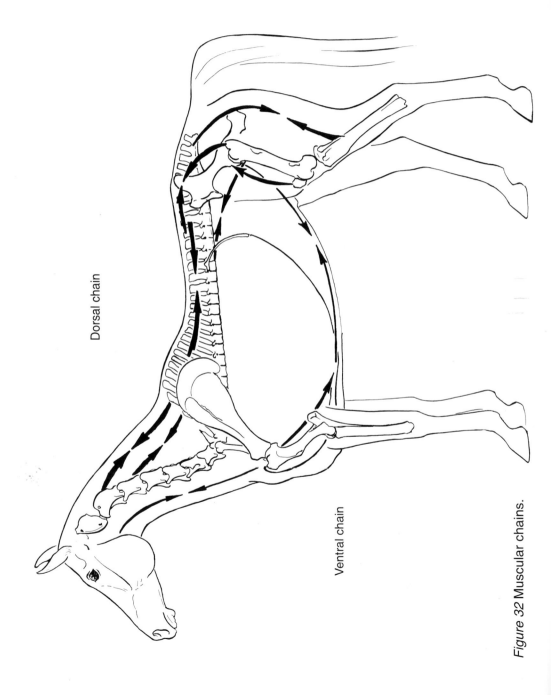

Dorsal chain

Ventral chain

Figure 32 Muscular chains.

having been poorly worked. Treatment of this area must follow that of the ventral chain, described next, and not the other way around.

2. VENTRAL CHAIN

2.1 Constituent parts

1. Cervical ventral muscles – flexors of the neck.
2. Abdominal muscles – flexors of the thoraco-lumbar spine, the lumbo-sacral and coxo-femoral joints.
3. Cranial femoral muscles – flexors of the hip.

2.2 Anchorage points
The abdominal section is formed by the stratification of several muscular groups which intersect with each other; it extends between the costo-xiphoid and pubic and inguinal points. The cervical section extends between the cephalic and sterno-costal points.

2.3 Action
The abdominal and cervical sections converge on the thoracic relay, forming a synergistic union. Looking again at Fig. 32 it is convenient to describe the dorsal and ventral chains in terms of two lines: 'top' and 'bottom', respectively. The 'bottom' line assists the 'top' line in all activity involving the lifting of the forelimbs. It acts as the 'floor' from which the dorsal and ischio-tibial muscular chains move the forelimbs, assisting the extension of the erector spinae muscles.This muscular synergy is fundamental to the support of the vertebral column as well as to the flexion involved in engagement. The dorsal chain needs to be relaxed if the ventral chain is to function effectively, and the trainer should pay close attention to to the abdominal muscles which form the abdominal 'girdle' during exercises. The cervical section works in synergy with the abdominal section. The pressure with which the horse engages with the bit indicates when it is placed under tension; this enhances lumbar flexion.

Exercises which bring about these biomechanical events appear to be particularly important in order to compensate for overwork which involves vertebral extension; young horses should also not be urged to raise their neck straight away. During sporting events or when in riding school, nimbleness of the forelimbs proceeds from the lowering of the haunches which is effected by tensing the 'bottom' line. It should not only be the result of lifting the neck brought about by accentuating the cervico-thoracic curve; this brings two muscular groups which are usually antagonistic but complementary (the cervical ventral and abdominal sections of the ventral chain) into opposition, and can cause artificial gaits and other locomotor problems.

3. EQUILIBRIUM
A point of equilibrium exists between the top/bottom (or extensor/flexor) groups, which is essential to all equitation. It cannot be achieved until the abdominal musculature is in the correct state of tonus. Unless the horse is relaxed and confident, successful work and the development of appropriate musculature cannot be undertaken; the dorsal chain will be predominant, locking the 'top' line and hindering amplitude of movement.

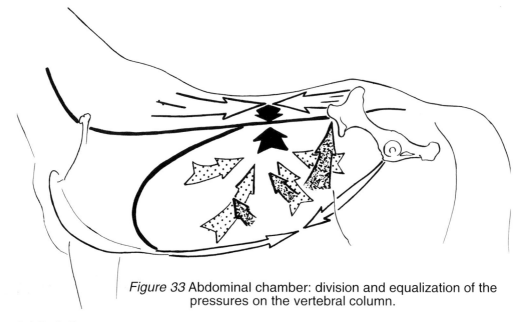

Figure 33 Abdominal chamber: division and equalization of the pressures on the vertebral column.

3.1 Pathology

As Busquet[1] has commented, the muscular chains possibly account for the recurrence of lesions, as each link in the chain is a potential 'fuse' which can blow when the circuit is placed under too much pressure. Movement within a healthy body is organized around the following principles – equilibrium, economy of effort and comfort. The muscular chains are no exception, creating a functional unity. Biomechanical disorders can break this unity, creating problems within the chain or at some distance from it as a result of myo-fascial connections.

3.2 Myo-fascial levels

Two aponeurotic layers extend dorsally and ventrally, holding the muscular masses of the chains in position. Each of these layers contains fibres which are woven together and criss-cross obliquely:

1. The dorsal layer envelops the dorsal chain, and is placed under tension by the thoracic serratus muscles. It extends from the coxo-femoral (hip) joint to the base of the neck.
2. The ventral layer acts as an extension to the oblique muscles in the abdomen; it is covered with a thick elastic lamina, the abdominal membrane, which plays an important, passive, role in holding the viscera and vertebral bridge in position.

(b) The concept of the abdominal 'chamber'

'Without abdominal muscles there is no back.'

1. DEFINITION

Contraction of the abdominal muscles against the resistance provided by the diaphragm causes pressures within the abdomino-pelvic cavity; this then becomes, in effect, an abdominal

[1] L. Busquet. *Traite d'osteopathie myotensive*. Tome 1, les chaines musculaires du tronc et de la colonne cervicale. Maloine.

pressure chamber. Pressures circulate within the chamber as shown in Fig. 33, with those transmitted by the viscera pushing against forces generated by the back. This action is reinforced by the remarkable way in which the muscles of the abdominal wall provide a system of 'stays' which support the intervertebral joints. The effectiveness of this support depends on the state of tonus of the muscles.

The vertebral column and the muscles of the trunk thus combine to form an anatomical 'ridge' or 'beam'. The 'grain' of this ridge is neutral, that is, its axis follows the path of least resistance, and does not diverge from that of the vertebral axis provided that the muscles involved in flexion and extension are in equilibrium.

2. APPLICATION

In human medicine the fundamental role played by the abdominal wall in the support of the lumbar spine has been emphasized frequently. The musculature of this 'girdle' is implicated in most cases of lumbago. In the Horse, the vertical forces exerted on the thoraco-lumbar bridge, which include pregnancy (gravity) and the weight of the rider, are at the root of many musculo-tendinous and osteo-articular problems. As in human medicine, therapy and prevention of vertebral problems begin with the reinforcement of the vertebral column's means of support. This involves looking at the response to the weight of the trunk and of the rider, working on posture and studying the way in which the hind limbs engage during exercise.

The muscular chains control lumbo-sacral and coxo-femoral flexion, and are thus involved in the system which connects support for the back with the engagement of the hind limbs. This system is the main focus for physiotherapeutic treatment as well as training programmes, and is one of the main preoccupations of riders and trainers.

3. SUMMARY

Fig. 34 illustrates the postural, gymnastic and therapeutic points which have been discussed so far. The key to the ensemble is the responsiveness of the ventral chain, which makes the following possible:

1. Antigravid thoraco-lumbar flexion.
2. Counterbalancing of the erector spinae muscles involved in extension; in particular, it contributes to recentering the 'ridge' so that it maintains its neutral axis, and relieves the forehand by its support of the thoraco-lumbar bridge.

2. FORELIMB

2.1 SURFACE ANATOMY (See Figs. 35 to 37)

2.2 JOINTS

In the Equidae, the joints of the limbs are limited to flexion and extension. Only the joints of the pelvic and pectoral girdles are able to execute lateral and rotary movements.

In the forelimbs, only the shoulder-joint allows *abduction* and *adduction* (respectively, movement away from and towards the median plane); examples include the lateral movements involved in work on two tracks. In all the other joints, rotary, lateral or sliding movements are exclusively passive; they occur when support is required or to provide cushioning to absorb shocks from irregularities in the ground. The more a joint is distal to these movements, the greater their amplitude. They cannot be evaluated clinically unless the limb is raised.

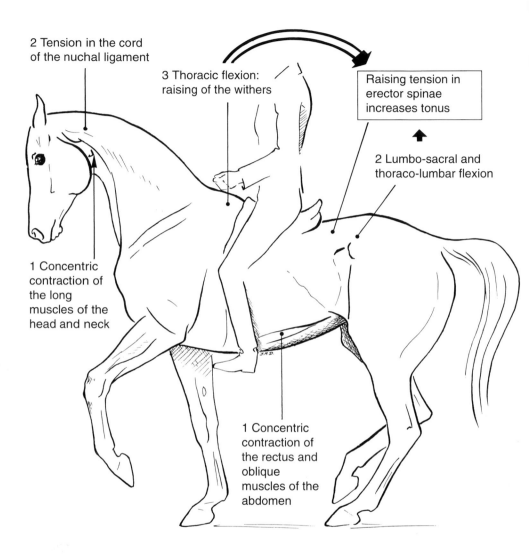

2 Tension in the cord
of the nuchal ligament

3 Thoracic flexion:
raising of the withers

Raising tension in
erector spinae
increases tonus

2 Lumbo-sacral and
thoraco-lumbar flexion

1 Concentric
contraction of
the long
muscles of the
head and neck

1 Concentric
contraction of
the rectus and
oblique
muscles of the
abdomen

Figure 34 Functioning as an ensemble, the muscles work together to accentuate
the curves in the vertebral column.

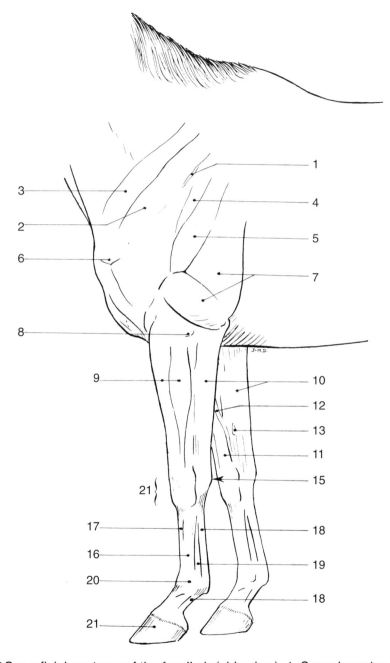

Figure 35 Superficial anatomy of the forelimb (side view). 1. Scapular spine.
2. Supraspinatus. 3. Subclavius. 4. Infraspinatus. 5. Deltoid. 6. Shoulder joint.
7. Triceps brachii. 8. Elbow joint. 9. Cranial antebrachial muscles. 10. Caudal
antebrachial muscles. 11. Radius. 12. Cephalic vein of the forearm. 13. Chestnut.
14. Knee joint. 15. Protuberance of the accessory carpal bone. 16. Metacarpal
bone. 17. Tendons of the digital extensor. 18. Tendons of the digital flexor.
19. Suspensor ligament of the pastern joint (3rd interosseous muscle).
20. Metacarpophalangeal joint. 21. Foot.

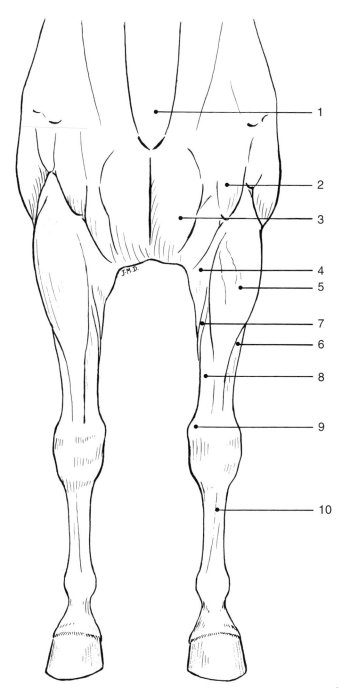

Figure 36 Superficial anatomy of the forelimb (frontal view). 1. Sternocephalic. 2. Brachiocephalic. 3. Descending pectoral. 4. Transverse pectoral. 5. Radial extensor of the carpus. 6. Dorsal digital extensor. 7. Cephalic vein of the forearm. 8. Radius. 9. Styloid process of the radius. 10. Dorsal tendon of the digital extensor.

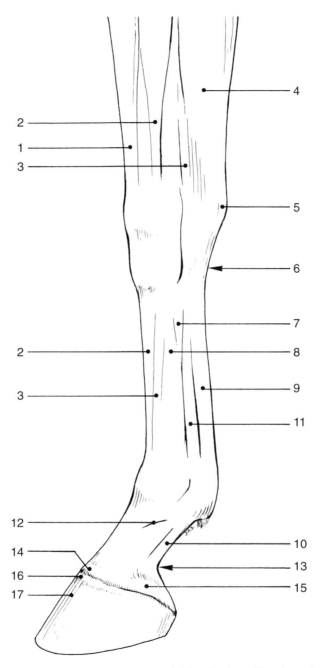

Figure 37 Superficial anatomy of the forelimb (side view). 1. Tendon of the radial extensor of the carpus. 2. Tendon of the common digital extensor. 3. Tendon of the lateral digital extensor. 4. Ulnaris lateralis. 5. Accessory carpal bone. 6. Fold of the knee. 7. Rudimentary lateral metacarpal bone. 8. Principal metacarpal bone. 9. Tendons of the deep and superficial digital flexors (perforans and perforatus). 10. Perforans tendon. 11. Suspensor ligament of the pastern (3rd interosseous muscle). 12. Attachment of suspensor ligament. 13. Fold of the pastern. 14. Coronary band. 15. Ungual cartilage. 16. Periople. 17. Hoof wall.

2.3 EXTRINSIC MUSCLES

Extrinsic muscles have insertions in areas outside of the member; in the case of the forelimbs, in the trunk, neck and head. They carry out two essential functions:

1. Support of the thorax in the area between the forelimbs and around the shoulders.
2. Coordination of the movements of the forelimbs during locomotion.

(a) Support of the thorax and forehand

This is the product of two powerful muscular 'corsets', one superimposed above the other (Fig. 38):

1. The *serratus* corset, formed by the cervical and thoracic ventral serratus.
2. The *pectoral* corset, formed by the ascending pectoral and subclavius.

Their effectiveness depends on the strength of the two muscular attachments (Fig. 39) which connect the forelimb to the trunk while allowing extensive mobility for the shoulder and arm. These are:

1. The dorsal attachment, which is secured by the trapezius, rhomboid and latissimus dorsi muscles.
2. The ventral attachment, which is formed by the descending and transverse pectoral muscles.

(b) Movements of the forelimb during locomotion

1. PROTRACTION AND RETRACTION

These movements are produced by the concentric contraction of composite muscle groups (Fig. 40).

Protraction describes the movement by which the horse extends the forelimb on the ground ahead of it. There are two groups of muscles involved, dorsal and ventral:

1. The dorsal group consists of the thoracic trapezius muscle and the caudal bundles of the ventral serratus; it draws the dorsal extremity of the scapula backwards.
2. The ventral group consists of the descending pectoral, brachiocephalic and omotransverse muscles; it draws the humerus and the ventral angle of the scapula forwards.

Retraction is the movement where the horse subsequently draws the limb back, producing propulsion. Again, two powerful groups of muscles are involved:

1. The dorsal group, consisting of the rhomboid, trapezius, cervical serratus and subclavius muscles.
2. The ventral group, consisting of the ascending pectoral and latissimus dorsi muscles.

2. ADDUCTION – ABDUCTION

During the various gaits, transverse movements of the limbs are never symmetrical; the intensity of action produced by each abductor and adductor muscle varies from one side to the other.

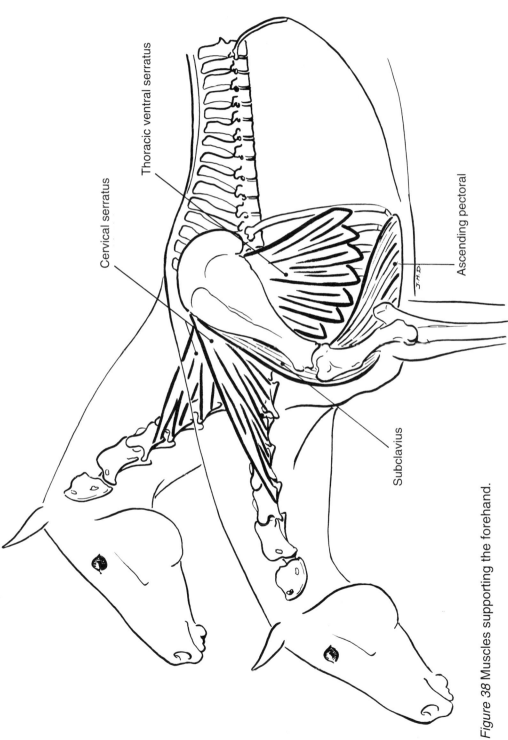

Thoracic ventral serratus

Cervical serratus

Ascending pectoral

Subclavius

Figure 38 Muscles supporting the forehand.

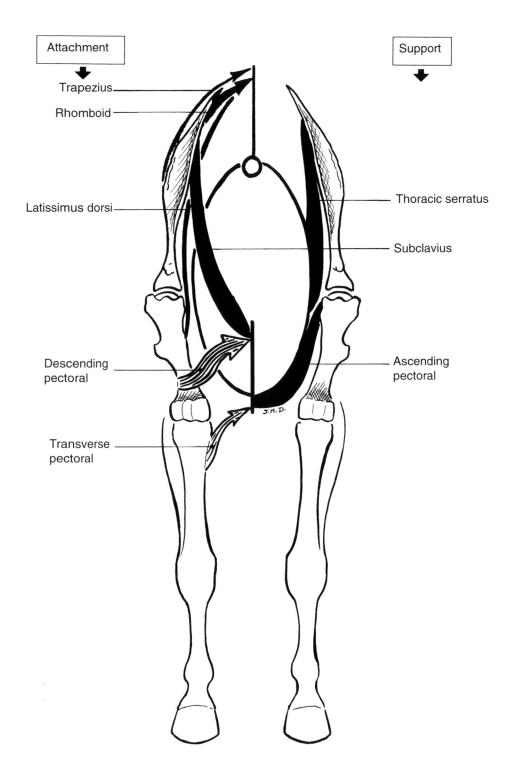

Figure 39 Muscles connecting the forelimb to the trunk and involved in supporting the forehand.

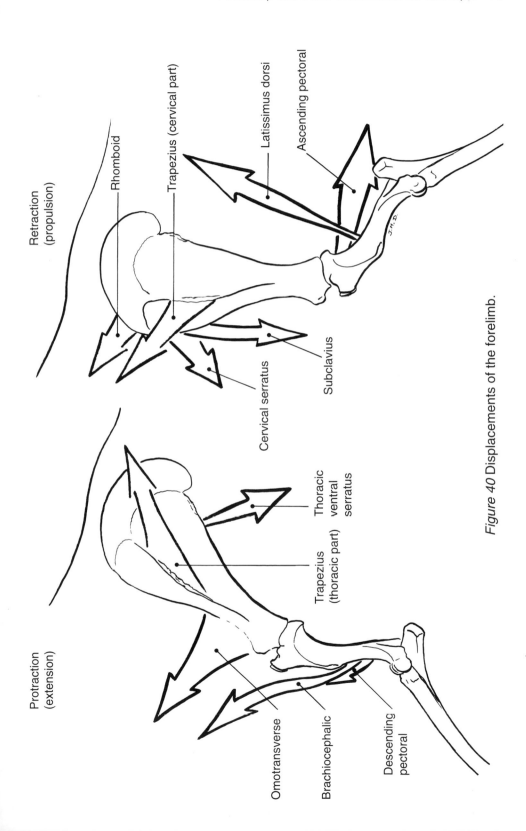

Retraction (propulsion)

Rhomboid

Trapezius (cervical part)

Latissimus dorsi

Ascending pectoral

Cervical serratus

Subclavius

Protraction (extension)

Thoracic ventral serratus

Trapezius (thoracic part)

Omotransverse

Brachiocephalic

Descending pectoral

Figure 40 Displacements of the forelimb.

1. *Adduction* (Fig. 41) is produced mainly by the descending, transverse and ascending pectoral muscles; adduction of the scapular-humeral joint is produced by the subscapularis.
2. *Abduction* (Fig. 42) is produced by muscles which are both extrinsic and intrinsic; the extrinsic muscles are trapezius and rhomboid, which draw the dorsal extremity of the scapula medially and effect the release of the shoulder joint. The intrinsic muscles are infraspinatus and deltoid, which are abductors of the shoulder joint.

2.4 INTRINSIC MUSCLES

In the Horse, three groups of muscles can be distinguished (although below the carpals there are no striated muscles at all). These are (Figs. 43, 44):

1. The muscles of the shoulder, which are monoarticular (i.e. involving a single joint).
2. The muscles of the arm, the most powerful of which are biarticular.
3. The muscles of the forearm, which are all multiarticular.

(a) Muscles of the shoulder
These mobilize the scapular-humeral joint exclusively. Functionally, they can be classified as:

1. Extensor (supraspinatus).
2. Flexors (deltoid and teres major).
3. Adductors (subscapularis and brachialis).
4. Abductors (infraspinatus and teres minor).

(b) Muscles of the arm
These produce all the movements of the elbow joint:

1. Flexors (biceps brachii and brachialis).
2. Extensors (triceps brachii – long, lateral and medial heads).
3. Tensor fasciae antebrachii.
4. Anconeus.

Two of these – biceps brachii and triceps brachii (long head) – are biarticular and bring together the joints of the shoulder and elbow. The former also acts as a support during scapular-humeral extension, while the latter supports flexion of the same joint.

(c) Muscles of the forearm
These extend along the pisiform, metacarpal and phalanx bones, attached by quite long tendons. Due to the mechanical specialization of the joints in the foot, they can be distinguished topographically and functionally. The cranial antebrachial muscles are the extensors of the carpus and digit. The most powerful – the radial extensor of the carpus – is equally a flexor of the elbow. The caudal antebrachial muscles are both flexors of the carpus and digits, and extensors of the elbow.

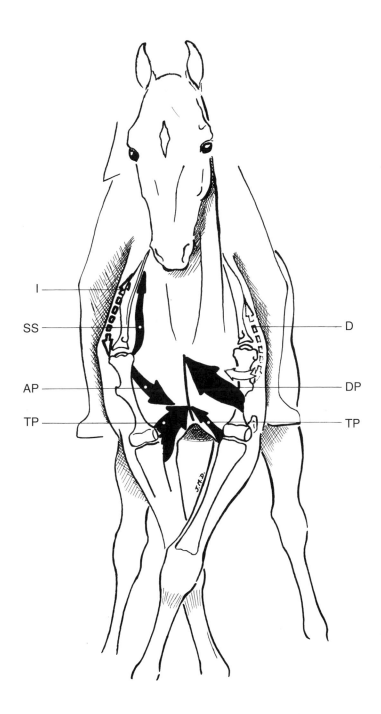

Figure 41 Muscular movements to produce adduction of the forelimbs.
Concentric contraction: DP, descending pectoral; TP, tranverse pectoral;
AP, ascending pectoral; SS, subscapularis.
Elongation: I, infraspinatus; D, deltoid.

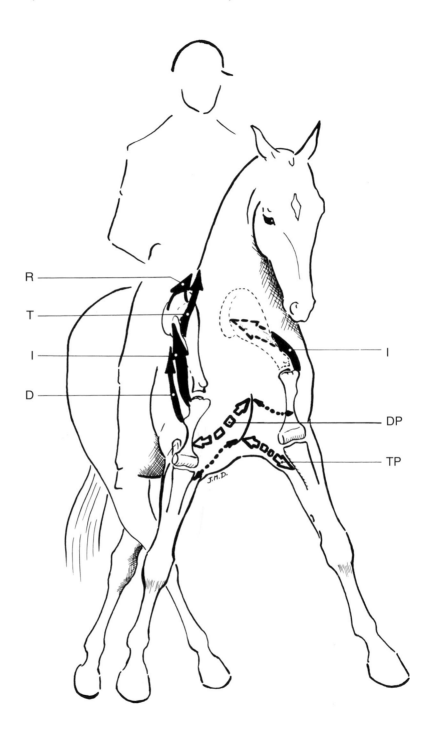

Figure 42 Muscular movements to produce abduction of the forelimbs.
Concentric contraction: I, infraspinatus; D, deltoid; R, rhomboid; T, trapezius.
Elongation: DP, descending pectoral; TP, transverse pectoral.

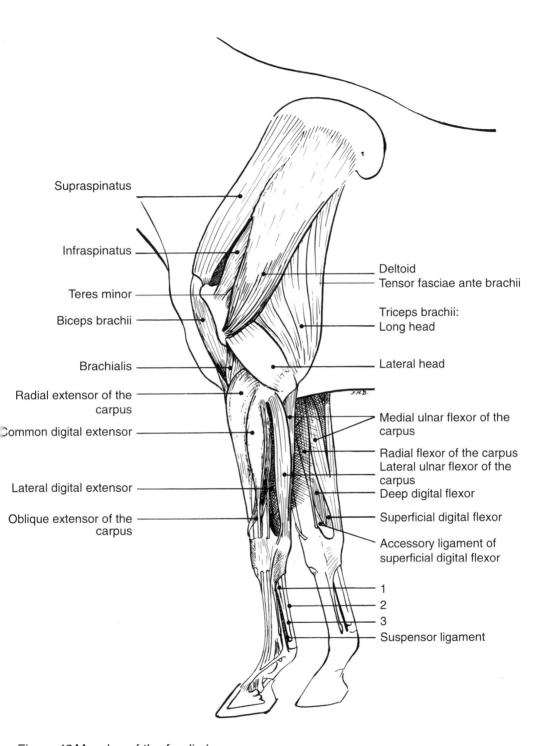

Supraspinatus

Infraspinatus

Teres minor

Biceps brachii

Brachialis

Radial extensor of the carpus

Common digital extensor

Lateral digital extensor

Oblique extensor of the carpus

Deltoid
Tensor fasciae ante brachii

Triceps brachii:
Long head

Lateral head

Medial ulnar flexor of the carpus

Radial flexor of the carpus
Lateral ulnar flexor of the carpus
Deep digital flexor

Superficial digital flexor

Accessory ligament of superficial digital flexor

1
2
3
Suspensor ligament

Figure 43 Muscles of the forelimb.
1. Accessory ligament of the deep digital flexor. 2. Tendon of the superficial digital flexor. 3. Tendon of the deep digital flexor.

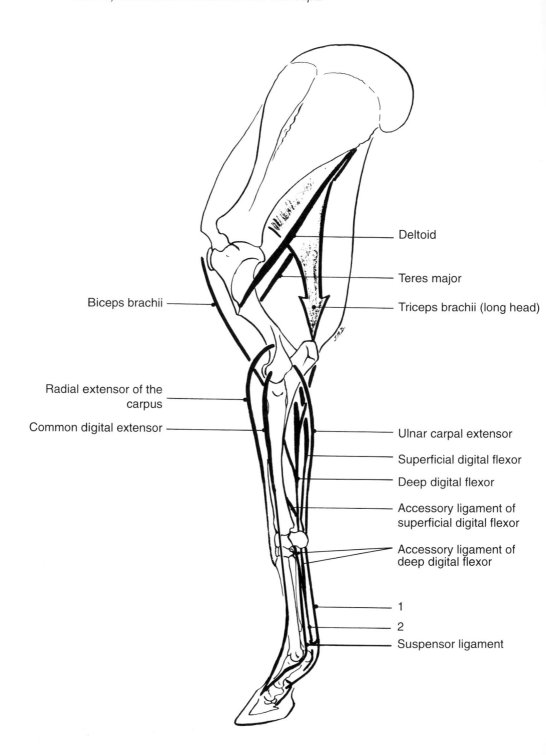

Figure 44 Muscles of the forelimb.
1. Tendon of the superficial digital flexor. 2. Tendon of the deep digital flexor.

1. CRANIAL ANTEBRACHIAL MUSCLES
Extensors of the carpus:

- Radial (also a support during flexion of the elbow).
- Oblique.

Extensors of the carpus and digit:

- Common digital.
- Lateral digital.

2. CAUDAL ANTEBRACHIAL MUSCLES
Flexors of the carpus:

- Lateral ulnar.
- Medial ulnar.
- Radial (large palmar).

Flexors of the digit:

- Superficial; extended by the perforatus tendon.
- Deep; extended by the perforans tendon.

It is important to emphasize that all the muscles of the forelimb work harmoniously together to produce locomotion. This is further helped by the way in which joints lock to prevent antagonistic muscle groups working against each other during extension. It is also remarkable that during propulsion, extension of the interphalangeal joints is a product of the contraction of flexors in the digit!

(d) Foot (carpus, metacarpus and digit)
This area is covered by fibrous structures. In addition to the tendons of the muscles mentioned earlier, there is the interosseous suspensor ligament, which plays a number of important supporting roles.

3. PELVIC LIMB

3.1 SURFACE ANATOMY
(Figs. 45, 46)

3.2 JOINTS
As with the thoracic limb, the joints of the pelvic limb are assigned to paramedian movements of flexion and extension. The coxo-femoral (hip) joint can only make it move in a partly lateral manner, as abduction is reduced by the presence of a supplementary ligament joined to the ligament attached to the head of the femur. Active mobilization of joints in the knee (stifle), hock and digit involves flexion and extension alone. All other lateral, rotary or sliding

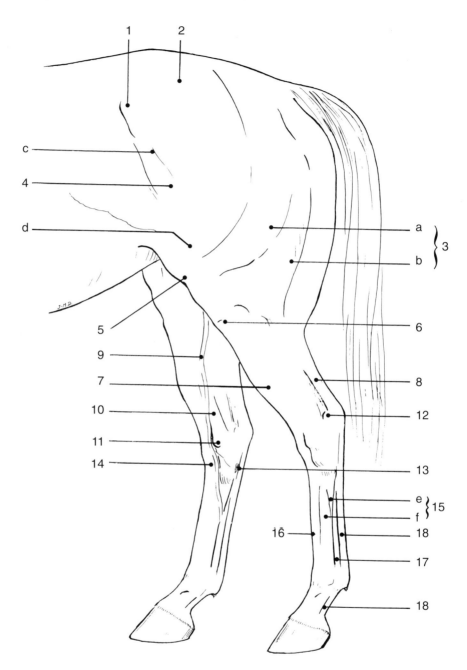

Figure 45 Superficial anatomy of the hind-limb (side view).
1. Ilium. 2. Middle gluteal. 3. Caudal femoral muscles: (a) gluteofemoral, (b) biceps femoris. 4. Cranial femoral muscles: (c) tensor fasciae latae, (d) quadriceps femoris. 5. Patella. 6. Tibial tuberosity. 7. Cranial muscles of the leg. 8. Hamstring (calcaneal tendon). 9. Median saphenous vein. 10. Tibia. 11. Medial-malleolus of the tibia. 12. Calcaneus. 13. Chestnut. 14. Point of the hock. 15. Cannon bone: (e) rudimentary lateral metatarsal, (f) third metatarsal. 16. Extensor tendons of the digit. 17. Suspensory ligament of the fetlock (3rd interosseous muscle). 18. Flexor tendons of the digit.

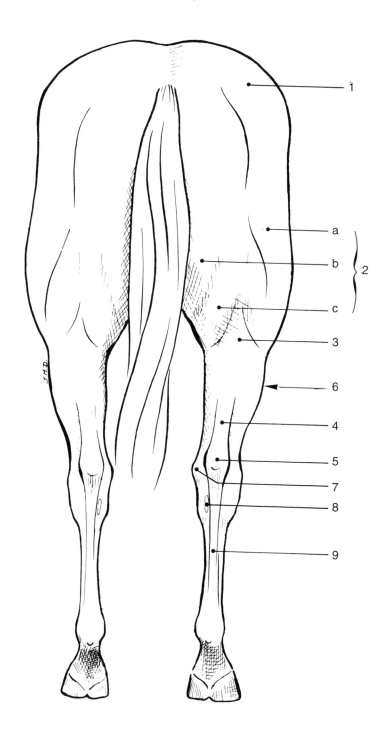

Figure 46 Superficial anatomy of the rump.
1. Middle gluteal. 2. Caudal femoral muscles (a) gluteobiceps,
(b) semimembranosus, (c) semitendinosus. 3. Gastrocnemius. 4. Hamstring.
5. Cap of the calcaneus. 6. Cranial muscles of the leg. 7. Medial-malleolus
of the tibia. 8. Chestnut. 9. Flexor tendons of the digit.

movements are passive, that is to say, they are only involved when support or cushioning is required. The movements of the digit and knee are of greater amplitude than those of the hock.

3.3 EXTRINSIC MUSCLES

With the pelvis closely connected to the vertebral column by the sacro-iliac joints, there is little diversification of the extrinsic musculature of the pelvic limb. The major muscle here is the iliopsoas, attached to the minor trochanter of the femur (Fig. 47), with two components, the iliacus and psoas major. It is a powerful flexor of the coxo-femoral joint, and is also an external rotator and adductor. Movement of the limb, which cannot take place without the involvement of this joint, is effected by the intrinsic muscles of the pelvis and thigh.

3.4 INTRINSIC MUSCLES

Using the same system of identification that was employed in the description of the thoracic limb, three groups can be distinguished by location and function (Fig. 48). These are:

1. The muscles of the pelvis, monoarticular with the exception of the middle gluteal.
2. The muscles of the thigh, which are mostly biarticular.
3. The muscles of the leg, which are all polyarticular except for the popliteus.

(a) Muscles of the pelvis
These are all involved in activating the coxo-femoral joint. The middle gluteal is also involved in extension of the lumbo-sacral and sacro-iliac joints. There are two groups which differ in their dimensions and functions:

1 THE GLUTEAL MUSCLES
The middle gluteal is by far the most powerful of the group (Fig. 49). It is covered by the superficial gluteal and hides the deep and accessory gluteal (Fig. 50). These muscles are primarily extensors, and to a lesser extent, abductors and internal rotators, of the coxo-femoral joint (Fig. 51).

2. THE DEEP PELVIC MUSCLES
These surround the coxo-femoral joint. While they are much less efficient physiologically than the gluteal muscles, they are involved in joint restraint, and in proprioception (i.e. they have a cybernetic role).

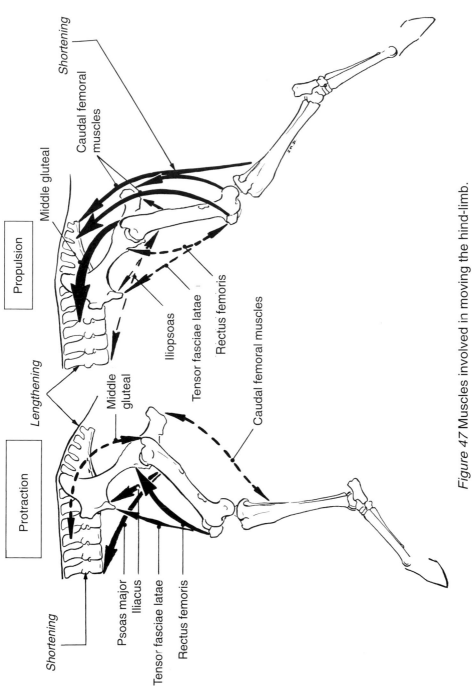

Figure 47 Muscles involved in moving the hind-limb.

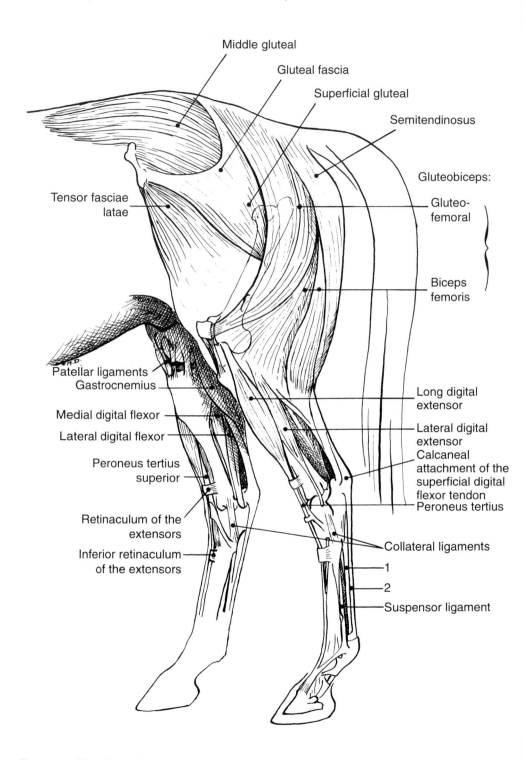

Figure 48 Muscles of the hind-limb (superficial level).
1. Tendon of the deep digital flexor. 2. Tendon of the superficial digtial flexor.

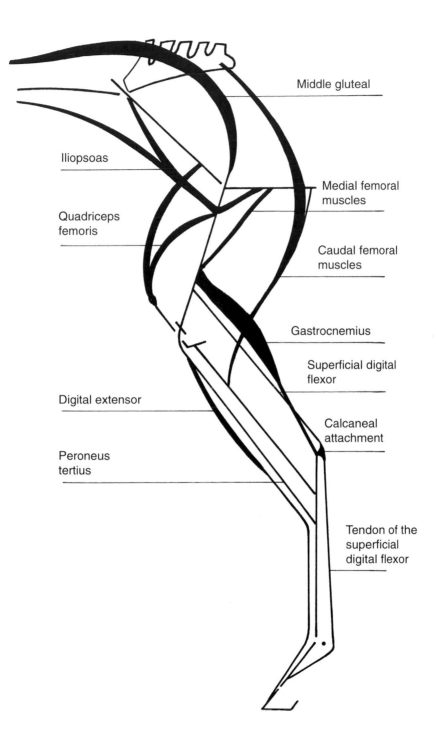

Figure 49 Muscular groups of the hind-limb.

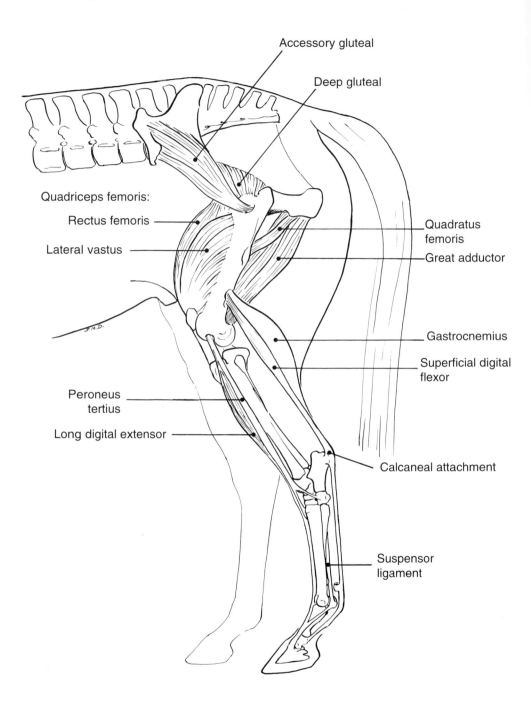

Figure 50 Muscles of the hind-limb (deep level).

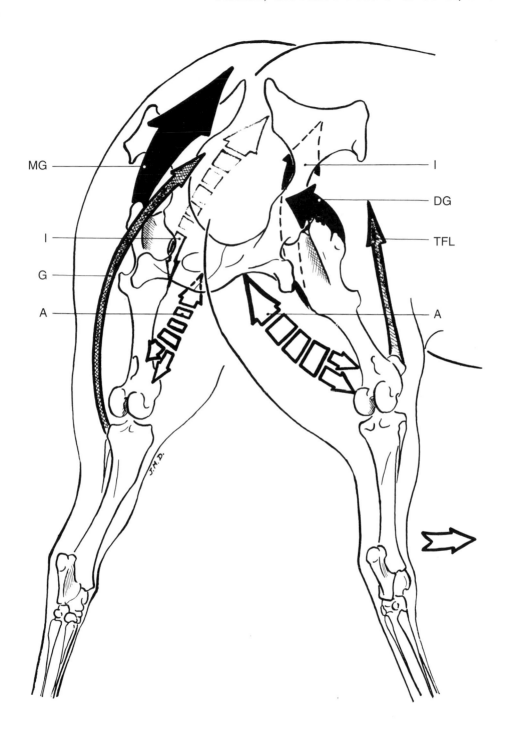

Figure 51 Muscles involved in the abduction of the hind-limbs.
Concentric contraction: MG, middle gluteal; DG, deep gluteal; G, gluteobiceps;
I, iliopsoas; TFL, tensor fasciae latae.
Elongation: A, adductors of the thigh; I, iliopsoas.

(b) Muscles of the thigh

These surround the femur, and can be divided by location and function into three groups:

1. CRANIAL FEMORAL MUSCLES

These large, powerful muscles, the quadriceps femoris, are primarily extensors of the knee. One of them, the rectus femoris, is also a flexor of the hip; this action is also the main role of the tensor fasciae latae.

2. CAUDAL FEMORAL MUSCLES

Two of these, the semitendinosus and biceps femoris, insert into the leg. The other two, the gluteo-femoral and semimembranosus, are attached to the area around the knee. These powerful muscles originate in the pelvis; they work synergistically with the gluteal muscles as extensors of the coxo-femoral joint, and with the quadriceps femoris as extensors of the knee in a supportive role. The biceps femoris and semitendinosus are also supportive flexors of the knee, this time working antagonistically against the quadriceps femoris

3. MEDIAN FEMORAL MUSCLES

These are arranged in two superimposed levels (Figs. 52, 53). The two superficial muscles, sartorius and gracilis, are flattened. The deep muscles, pectineus and adductor (great and short), are thick. They are all adductors of the coxo-femoral joint and for this reason are antagonist to the gluteal muscles. The sartorius is a flexor and external rotator of the joint. The great adductor is also a powerful extensor and internal rotator. Pectineus also provides articular support.

(c) Muscles of the leg

There is a pronounced mechanical specialization of joints of the hock and digit, imposed by function and location.

1. CRANIAL MUSCLES

Two of these are exclusively flexors of the tibio-talus joint. These are are the cranial tibial and peroneus tertius muscles. The latter, which is completely fibrous in the Horse, is also called the femoro-metatarsal cord. The other two muscles are extensors of both the metacarpo-digital and interphalangeal joints: these are the long and lateral digital extensors, which converge on the same tendon on the anterior face of the cannon.

2. CAUDAL MUSCLES

These fall into two groups, superficial (1) and deep (2):

1. The superficial group consists of the gastrocnemius (extensor of the hock) and the superficial digital flexor. The latter, which is also completely fibrous in the horse, is responsible for both the support and flexion of the fetlock and proximal interphalangeal joints.
2. The deep group consists of the medial and lateral deep digital flexor and caudal tibial muscles, as well as the popliteus (a flexor and internal rotator of the knee). The former are flexors of the metacarpo-digital and interphalangeal joints and responsible for the extension of the latter during propulsion. They have a minor role in acting on the tibio-talus joint.

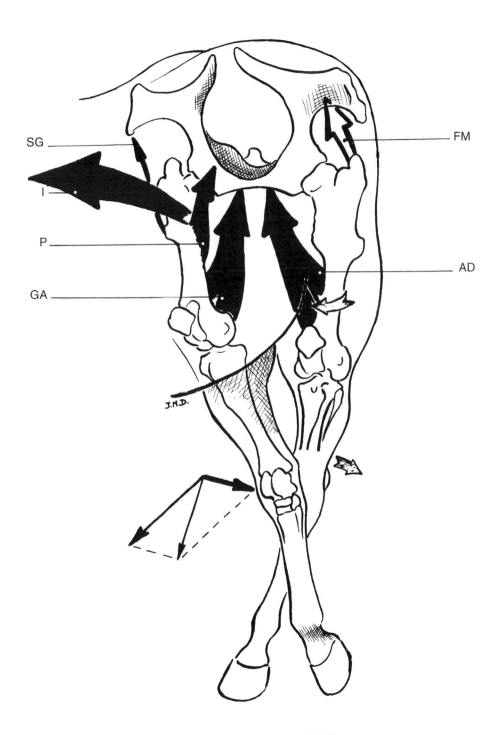

Figure 52 Adduction of the hind-limbs during lateral diplacements.
GA, great adductor; I, iliopsoas; P, pectineus; SG, superficial gluteal; MG, middle
gluteal.

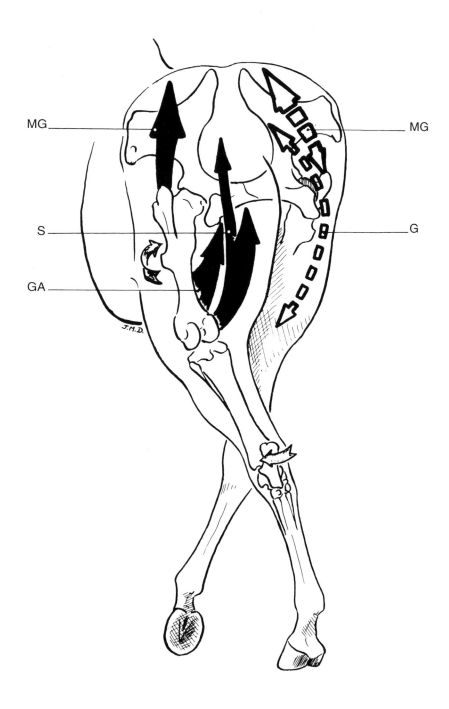

Figure 53 Adduction of the hind-limbs during lateral displacements.
Concentric contraction: GA, great adductor; S, semimembranosus.
Elongation: MG, middle gluteal; G, gluteobiceps.

3. RECIPROCITY WITHIN THE SYSTEM

Fig. 54 illustrates diagramatically the remarkable system which is worked by two tendinous cords – the peroneus tertius (femoro-metatarsal) and superficial digital flexor, which extends to the middle phalanx. Together with the skeletal ridges to which the tendons are attached, this system intermeshes the femoro-tibial, tibio-tarsal and metacarpo-digital joints.

From a resting position, flexion of the knee draws on the proximal insertion of the peroneus tertius, causing flexion of the hock. The calcaneus acts on the superficial digital tendon, causing it to recoil, inducing flexion of the metacarpo-digital joint.

The femoro-tibial extension brought about by the powerful femoral muscles draws on the proximal insertion of the superficial digital flexor, which transmits its force along the calcaneus, provoking the extension of the hock. The force of the returning calcaneus on the cord allows the extension of the digit. The system continually regulates the biomechanics of the pelvic limb, except during a few extreme postures or lively gaits.

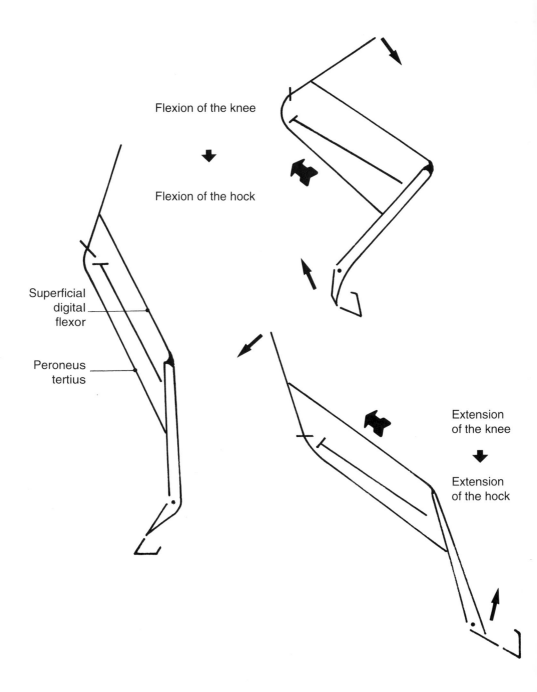

Figure 54 System of reciprocal interconnection of the movements of the knee and hock joints.

3 Synthesis and Applications

1. THE HORSE'S BACK REFLECTS EMOTIONAL AND PSYCHOMOTOR DISTURBANCE

In comparison to the human back, which is a vertical column, that of the horse resembles a horizontal bridge, stretched between the scapular and pelvic girdles. Although it is the limbs which provide propulsion, it is the back which is the crucial anatomical component of equine biomechanics, and which is the true source of motion, equilibrium and coordination. Impulsion produced by excessive activity on the part of the limbs may be mistaken for genuine mastery of the flexible, cadenced and strong movements associated with lumbar flexion, but is no substitute for it. Achieving vertebral mobility requires that the rider:

1. Finds the cadence that best corresponds to the individual horse's style, for each horse develops according to a particular tempo which allows it ease of movement and corresponds to its physical structure and temperament.
2. Establishes a relationship based on mutual confidence, creating a lack of inhibition in movement which transmits itself to the back.

In the horse, as with human beings, where the process is well understood and plays a large part in everyday medical general practice, emotional and psychomotor problems reveal themselves in the back. When we are under constant tension, and stressed and fatigued as a result, it is not uncommon to see the symptoms of a vertebral pathology. The Celts, who were afraid that the sky would fall on their heads, walked around with their necks hunched between their shoulders. This symbolic gesture finds its present day counterpart in the way we tense the muscles of the neck and spine when we are anxious.

The psychological aspect is thus fundamental, reflecting the 'top'/'bottom' line duality mentioned in the previous chapter. There is a point of biomechanical and psychological equilibrium which is reached when there is harmony between propulsion (top line/resistance and refusal) and flexion (bottom line/yielding, relaxation and acquiescence). At this point independence and submission, refusal and acquiescence, meet and balance each other.

Physiotherapy cannot be contemplated without a prior understanding of the sensory and instinctive nature of the horse. The sensory nature reveals itself in way the horse responds both to us and to its immediate environment; its instinctive nature deals with the world of emotional response and communication that we share in common. The true horseman will make himself familiar with both of them. Being on good terms with one's horse manifests itself in sound and unrestricted movement; a poor relationship reveals itself, at the competitive level, in movements which are hesitant and timorous.

1.1 THREE FUNDAMENTAL APPROACHES TO THE TREATMENT AND CARE OF THE BACK

(a) Counter the instinctive lifting and extension of the neck and head

Working in this way permits the interspinous spaces to open, develops the musculature of the flexors and lengthens the paravertebral muscles causing them to relax as a consequence. It strengthens the 'bottom' line.

(b) Engage the muscles involved in impulsion progressively and in stages

It is gentler on the horse to not raise the head until the final stages of exercise, when the abdominal muscles are sufficiently toned to maintain lumbar flexion.

(c) Reinforce the point of equilibrium

This will take two or three years of work on the 'top' and 'bottom' lines so that they work together harmoniously. This will result in nimbleness and an enhanced equilibrium – what in automotive terms might be described as a shorter 'turning circle'.

2. ENGAGEMENT AND RELAXATION

2.1 WORKING ON ENGAGEMENT AT THE TROT AND GALLOP

Engagement involves two axes: the coxo-femoral joint and lumbo-sacral hinge joint. The weight of the rider hinders lumbo-sacral flexion. When working with the young horse, it is therefore appropriate to develop engagement gradually, in two stages. During the first stage, which takes several months, work concentrates on obtaining excellent coxo-femoral mobility. This is achieved by working at gaits which are lively but balanced, not rushed. The abdominal muscles are also involved actively, but care is taken to work isotonically, to avoid shortening the muscle fibres. This having been accomplished, the second stage involves actively encouraging dorso-lumbar flexion by working isometrically, so that the fibres of the muscles of the abdomen and abdominal girdle are shortened deliberately. At the trot, the abdominal girdle is directly involved in isometric maintenance of the abdominal floor. Its involvement sets in motion the active phase of muscular shortening which brings about dorso-lumbar flexion and enhances engagement and collection.

When this has been achieved the rider feels, as the expression goes, the 'loins' of the horse 'pass under the saddle'. The stride becomes cadenced and lighter and the horse's posture improves. For the horse, this active participation of the abdominal flexors requires intense effort. In the young horse it may be the source of fatigue and even cause myositis of the iliopsoas muscle. It is therefore desirable that a good part of the work takes place out of doors, so that walking up and down slopes will help tone the abdominal musculature. It is also important that the work in this area is 'little and often' rather than concentrated in sessions which are less frequent.

At the gallop, with a balanced gait, flexion of the hip normally involves lumbar flexion. The abdominal muscles contract concentrically, with one side or other of the oblique muscles predominating. This explains, amongst other things, the difficulty of executing the counter, or false, gallop, which requires the shortening of the oblique muscles while the rectus and iliopsoas simultaneously maintain the tilt of the pelvis and the flexion of the hip. This is why a young horse needs to have developed a strong abdominal girdle before beginning this type of exercise. Without it, a counter-gallop with a rigid and painful top line will be the result. Too many horses trot and gallop in this over-economical and defensive stance, which produces artificial movement in the front and rigidity in the rear. Developing the young horse for athletic performance involves creating a programme which is measured and carefully thought out before one begins specialized movements. Time spent away from competition can cause one to forget previous experience and the principle of progressivity.

It is worth reiterating at this stage two fundamental rules:

1. *'No abdominals, no back'*. Sound movement proceeds from a strong back, and a strong back from strong abdominal muscles.
2. *Engagement is the only way of exercising the horse without making it suffer.*

2.2 PATHOLOGY OF THE BACK: PREVENTING INJURY

As they occur in almost all the disciplines, common causes of vertebral problems include:

1. Premature attempts to perform specialized movements.
2. Inadequate or faulty loosening-up exercises.
3. Predominance of the extensors of the back over the abdominal muscles.

To correct these faults, or better still to avoid them, the following steps need to be taken:

1. Train the young horse gradually and wait for it to exhibit, of its own accord, aptitude for a specialized discipline.
2. Never begin a training session without warming up.
3. Combine mobilization of the back with work on a slope which develops dorsal, lumbar and sacral suppleness.

2.3 SHOULDER-IN AND SHOULDER-FORE

The technique of 'shoulder-in', as recommended by the famous instructor La Guérinière[1], marked a new stage in the athletic training of the horse. He discovered the merits of lumbo-abdominal flexion while drawing the shoulder in; the technique shortens the fibres in the abdominal muscles, predominantly the internal oblique, and, as with all abdominal therapy, is very useful as a means of preventing and treating vertebral problems.

He also remarked on the risks that riders take by bending the horse's neck before impulsion: "if a horse should happen to hold back, the lesson should be discontinued for a while and replaced by an extended and vigorous trot".

Steinbrecht was equally responsible for developing the concept of freedom of movement prior to the horse being made to undertake the 'next step'. As the short-bodied horses of the 18th century became a thing of the past, he understood that shoulder-in must be preceded by shoulder-fore if long backs were to be made supple in the most effective way. For the longer back, strengthening of the abdominal girdle must be carried out sensitively for it to be biomechanically effective.

[1] La Guérinière. *Ecole de cavalerie*. Editions des 4 Seigneurs, Grenoble, 1973.

Another commentator, Handler-Lessing from Vienna, noticed that:

"Horses with long and weak backs have a tendency to sink beneath a load, so that the weight of the rider is supported by the vertebral column rather than by the muscles. The horse attempts to escape the resultant pain by trying to 'outrun' its burden; the hindlimbs move out of sequence, further exasperating the concavity of the back; the head and the neck are lifted, and the final result is the horse resisting all direction maintained by tensioning the reins".[1]

The shoulder-fore technique is well adapted to physical preparation for shoulder-in for two reasons:

1. Impulsion proceeds directly, allowing lumbo-abdominal flexion.
2. It allows extensive inward curvature, enhancing mobility.

2.4 RELAXATION

A movement achieves maximum effect when it encounters no resistance or opposition; 'top/bottom' line antagonism must be avoided. The initial target is thus relaxation rather than coordination. Starting with relaxation, easy and pain-free movement is ensured by adhering to the following practices:

(a) Demarcate the gaits
Through relaxation, the joints are allowed to achieve full amplitude of movement. Regularity and cadence calm the horse and encourage it to participate fully. Movement which is full, regular, relatively slow but full of energy can then be developed. It is important that cadence is not changed when the transition stage is reached.

(b) Maintaining the gaits
An advanced posture used in dressage, which cannot be used with very young horses, this does not become apparent until the abdominal musculature is sufficiently developed. A reasonable time to start working with a horse would be at the end of its fourth year; before then, it is not worth risking damage to the cartilages in the joints (the hocks in particular).

2.5 WORK ON TWO TRACKS

No lateral work of this nature should be undertaken prematurely, before the prior development of lumbar flexion. If it is, there is a risk of locking 'top' line musculature, hampering flexion and resulting in movements which are overextended, rather than in engagement and support. Work on two tracks while thus disengaged leads to paravertebral muscular resistance with the following pathological results: resistance → contraction of the back → disobedience → uncoordinated movement.

[1] Handler-Lessing. *La haute Ecole espagnole de Vienne*. Albin Michel.

2.6 CONCLUSION: KNOWLEDGE AND LISTENING

For the rider, analytical understanding of the movements of the horse proceeds from following these two dicta:
1. Know the biomechanical rules and work with them.
2. Become one with the horse ('centaur yourself', to employ the charming French expression), so that your body responds to the subtle signs which emanate from its locomotion; these will provide the true guide to selecting the appropriate exercises to perform.

Training the equine athlete according to our own programmatic notions rather than according to its innate biomechanical disposition is surely wrong. If there is a great deal of vertebral pathology, its causes must be sought not only in the weight of the rider and overspecialized movements, but also in our lack of listening. If a horse could express itself as the human athlete does, it would inform us of its muscular contractions, stiffness and lumbago; as in human medicine, therefore, it is important to interrupt training for treatment. Clearly, when a human athlete does not stop training at the first sign of tendinitis or lumbago, the underlying problems which are momentarily obscured will lead to something more serious.

It is therefore important to listen to the horse, to observe it as it enters its box in order to determine the source of its aches from the previous day's exercises, and to watch its initial movements. In this way its future health will be safeguarded.

3. TEN ADDITIONAL CRITERIA FOR EXERCISE

Several criteria need to be taken into consideration when directing work for a horse:

1. Gait
2. Amplitude of movement
3. Impulsion
4. Speed, including resistance and endurance
5. Cadence
6. Frequency of work and rest periods
7. Weight, both with and without rider
8. Resistance or cooperation (hyper- or hypotonia: feeding problems)
9. Type of terrain (hard, soft)
10. Plane of work (flat, inclined)

Each of these must be carefully worked out in relation to the horse's age and state of preparation.

4. EXERCISE ON A SLOPING PLANE

Demarcate a circle which is 15 to 20 meters in diameter; in half of it create a variation in level of approximately 1.5 m. The work is performed on the lunge, so that the back is free and not bearing any weight. The object of the exercise is to re-educate the back; there are two stages, descent and ascent, and the following muscle groups are involved:

1. *Descent.* Eccentric work on the abdominal muscles (the effort involved in braking on a downward slope) and hip flexors;

2. *Ascent.* Synergistic and concentric work on the extensors of the hip and back (gluteal and paravertebral muscles).These muscles work concentrically during propulsion.

The main focus of work during the ascent is on the execution of propulsion when the 'top' line is extended and slightly open, and the nose is lowered. A row of cavalettis spaced 1.2 m apart in the flat part of the circle encourages cadence and moderates the length of stride. Horses familiar with the exercise may, at the end of the ascent, be encouraged to jump a cross-piece 50 cm high. If they show little aptitude for the exercise, attaching reins will serve no purpose. However, one can provide light assistance by using a chambon with a rubber attachment.

The cadence, at the trot, must be slow and deliberate. Initially, the exercises should last less than 15 minutes on each rein, progressively building up to 20 or 30 minutes. A maximum of two or three sessions per week is recommended. The exercise has the particular virtue of developing the vertebral-abdominal relationship, and helps correct problems caused by overspecialized movements. Improvements are soon seen in horses which have weak backs and poor muscular strength and propulsion. The system is illustrated in Fig. 55.

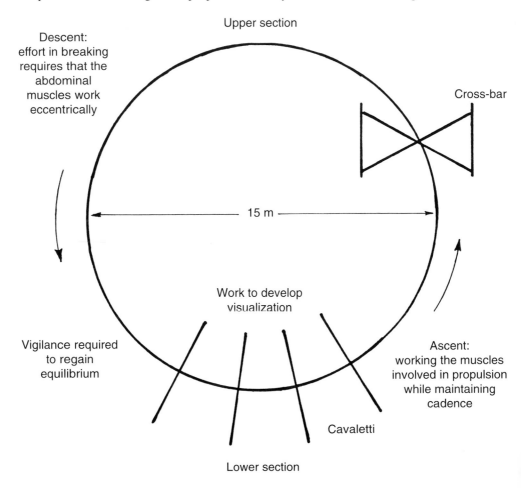

Figure 55 Work on an inclined plane.

PART TWO

1 General Introduction

The human athlete has no problem in describing precisely any muscular or articular problems he may be experiencing. Most of these are swiftly resolved by the rapid administration of therapy. His equine counterpart is no less subject to problems with muscles and joints, but the initial symptoms are often hidden, causing delay in the provision of care required to prevent more serious problems developing.

However, a sensitive and vigilant rider can detect signs of problems at their inception. The horse's initial movements in the box, or during the course of a training session, will reveal to the attentive trainer evidence of stiffness, lack of suppleness, nervousness, even resistance to certain commands. This is in sharp contrast to those who make their horse work immediately after leaving the box, as though it could move straight from the bedroom to running a 110 metre hurdle race. Not surprisingly, in these circumstances the horse will quickly start to suffer from tendinitis, many kinds of myalgia, and lumbar and other dorsal problems.

Another cause of many biomechanical problems is specialization in a particular discipline, which causes the same muscles and joints to be used repeatedly. As in human sports medicine, specific pathologies become apparent, but human athletes, with their greater awareness of health, can compensate for these problems, develop preventive measures, and can request rapid medical treatment.

1. THE HORSE IN COMPETITION; ATHLETICISM AND SUFFERING

From the moment that training for competition begins, most horses suffer. For them, competition is essentially traumatic and physiologically unnatural. During the course of obstacle jumping competitions, their cartilages and spinous processes are subjected to repeated shocks and minor traumas as they land following a jump and as a result of using artificial gaits. Conficts in engagement and collection become apparent in dressage. These mini-traumas often pass unnoticed in the young horse, but they have a cumulative effect. Bone growth is seldom taken into account, and excessive sporting activity by the colt will lead to pathologies which will reveal themselves later in life. Growth cartilages are situated in the areas around the joints (Fig. 56), and undergo pressures from traction and constraints from compression.

Traumas often pass unnoticed, but can cause creeping necrosis and are the source of arthrosis and arthritis in the articular cartilages, affecting the epiphyses as well as the apophyses. Fatigue resulting from overtraining also has a negative impact on the effectiveness of the synovial membranes, resulting in capsular distension (windgalls).

These cartilages are involved in the growth process as the horse grows taller; damage to them can thus distort the process of ossification, causing modifications in the shape and length of the bone, as well as epiphysary deformation, a cause of arthrosis.

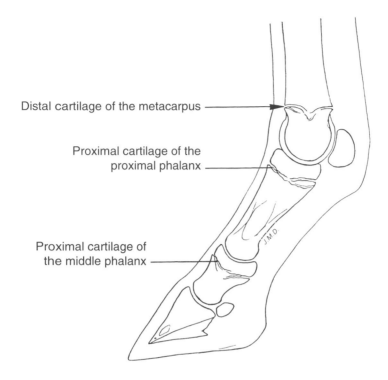

Distal cartilage of the metacarpus

Proximal cartilage of the
proximal phalanx

Proximal cartilage of
the middle phalanx

Figure 56 Drawing adapted from a radiographic image of growth cartilages in a foal
23 days old.

2. DEVELOPMENT AND BIOMECHANICAL ADAPTATION OF THE JOINT IN THE YOUNG HORSE

Cushioning is the first stage of absorbing the shock wave generated by pressure. In judo, striking the hand against the floor is intended to anticipate and absorb the shock wave before the body itself hits the floor. Without this technique the practitioner, or judoka, would have a short career in the sport. The horse, like the judoka, hits the ground with the forelimb; however, the iron shoe and the fact that the forelimb does not roll with the impact means that the shock is carried in virtually a straight line through the foot, knee and shoulder and thence to the spine. The trainer should therefore look closely at the quality of terrain: a hard surface risks damage to bones and joints, while a soft and deep surface risks damage to tendons, ligaments and muscles.

It is important to find a surface which is somewhere between the two. Above all, lengthy trotting on tarmac and landing on hard ground after a jump should be avoided, and frequent rest stops made. A young horse's first training sessions should have a rest period every 5 minutes. Examples of the way to apportion activity might be as follows: 3 periods at the trot for each period at the gallop; period of jumping followed by rest.

3. MASTERY OF LOCOMOTION

From the first session the aim must be to find and work with the horse's natural cadence. Each horse has its own tempo which must be respected; the discovery of this rhythm, at both the trot and gallop, leads to equilibrium and to sound and economical movement.

At this time, and taking care to remain on good terms with the horse, the trainer must make it accustomed to hearing and obeying orders, in particular:

1. Moving forwards and in reverse (braking and accelerating).
2. Moving sideways (incurvation and flexion).

It is desirable to make warming-up exercises follow precise geometric patterns; this will help prepare the horse at this initial stage to coordinate its gestures.

Walking restores calm and provides the opportunity to return to movements which were incompletely understood or poorly executed the first time. It also allows one to assess the confidence of the horses's comportment, and leads naturally to returning to the gallop and stretching exercises in work on two tracks.

4. JUMPING

The young horse should not be introduced directly to jumping; instead, during the course of a dressage session and then only if it is ready, it may be placed in front of an obstacle. For optimum performance of both horse and rider, the following objectives must be set:

For the horse:

1. Training in movement which is not physically overtaxing.
2. Introduction to a variety of experiences – colour, sequence and shape – during the course of work.
3. Frequent rest periods to help provide calm.
4. Treatment to regulate tonus if there is evidence of disturbance (e.g. anxiety or sluggishness).
5. Setting the appropriate height for an obstacle. This can be significant for a four year old, and should be no higher than 1 to 1.2 m; however, a well thought-out jump which is 1.2 m high is less dangerous than one of 80 cm which has been poorly executed as a result of loss of cadence and haste, or which is the product of the rider's demanding that the horse accomplish something before it is ready to do so.
6. Provision of adequate warm-up periods; regulation of sessions – two a week, 25 to 30 jumps per session, on suitable terrain to help prevent cumulative damage from mini-traumas.

For the rider:

1. Attention to be paid to one's own level of tonus, a factor which is crucial to both success and failure.
2. Remember that the horse is always aware of your emotional state and level of aggression.
3. A great competitor is always in control of his emotions and never lets himself get involved in disputes with judges.

4. The horse's back, which governs cadence and equilibrium, is a two-way street, not only transmitting the horse's emotional condition to the rider, but also transmitting that of the rider to the horse.

5. PROBLEMS CAUSED BY RIDING SCHOOL

One often finds the young horse being expected to attain standards of behaviour and physical prowess which would be considered inconceivable for a human being. These expectations bear no relationship to its stage of biomechanical development, and manifest in such practices as forcing it to adopt an unnaturally high position of the neck and poll, working on two tracks before the horse has acquired lateral and antero-posterior flexibility, and overriding cadence in order to make it perform continuous diagonals at the trot.

In these circumstances, the back becomes slack, or rather, it never reaches the optimum level of strength and flexibility; the hocks also reveal evidence of misuse. More importantly, there is a risk of neglecting to diversify work and employ stretching exercises in order to compensate for working excessively at collection. The result is hypertonia in the back, spasms and resistance arising from chronic lumbar problems and tired hocks.

2 Methods and Techniques

1. MASSAGE

1.1 PHYSIOLOGY OF THE SKIN

(a) Respiratory role
The skin is involved in respiration; the proportion of output for which it is responsible is between 0.5 and 0.8% of that provided by the lungs.

(b) Secretory role
There are several types of sweat which originate from different glands and which arise in response to various physiological and psychological causes. In both the Horse and Man, there are a greater number of sweat glands than in other mammals. In the Horse, sweat is acid and plays the following roles:

1. Thermal regulation.
2. Maintaining the suppleness of the skin.
3. Detoxification – elimination of toxins produced endogenously, arising from diet, fatigue and stress.

There is a constant minimal level of sweating, produced in periodic waves; in the Horse there are one or two of these waves each minute. When it is physically fatigued or emotionally stressed, sweating increases to reach its maximum level, remaining there until the recovery stage. Odours vary according to the composition of the sweat – water, dry matter, organic substances, minerals.

Odour is linked to sex and age; foals of both sexes have a fresh odour that is descibed as being 'milky', even after weaning. Males have a strong and musky odour, while mares in heat produce an odour that stallions can recognize as far away as 300 meters. The following associations between odour and temperament have been described: cold = lethargic; fresh = sanguine; pungent = spirited; peppery = choleric.

(c) Sensory role
The skin is richly innervated. It is an immense, extended nervous receptor, with freely branching terminations in the dermis and hypodermis. There are synaptic connections between the sensory receptors in the skin and deeply situated organs which permit cutaneo-muscular therapeutic treatment, such as reflex massage of an organ via cutaneous stimulation.

(d) Emotional role

According to Prof. Jean de Goldfiem[1], emotion is a cortical-thalamic-hypothalamic event, which, in the Horse, appears to be the source of bio-electrical activity in the skin; it can thus be recorded on an electroencephalogram (EEG) or electrodermagram.

1.2 INTRODUCTION TO MASSAGE

Massage must be a living experience; this means that it must be a source of perception, a means of exploring via the fingertips the painful muscle as it tenses and relaxes. It is not simply an action, but a means of therapeutic communication, where awareness is the product of the dialogue between an organ in pain and the hand which detects that pain and removes it. It is impossible to heal with one's hands if the desire to comfort is not also there. Healing requires total concentration, being alone with the horse, preferably within its box or in some other quiet place. While the sensitive points are being searched for, the horse will reveal its reactions through many movements or attitudes – looking towards the masseur, tension and relaxation. These constitute the language of the method.

Massage is a process of evolution. The next day different levels of tension may appear; every day reveals a new situation on the road to recovery.

The bulk and weight of a horse would appear to dictate that initial manipulations be deep and powerful; in fact, the same progression and sensitivity should be used as when practising massage on a human being. Massage movements should go with the lay of the hair, sometimes transversely, but never counter. Circular movements around a cramped muscle, for example, are made by working the fingers together as a solid unit on the skin. When using the flexed elbow to massage the muscles around the vertebrae, the flat part at the inferior extremity of the humerus rather than the point itself should be used. Movements should follow the direction of the muscular fibres, or be transverse to it. Using these techniques one can produce a stimulating as well as a therapeutic massage.

1.3 TECHNIQUE

Each level of contact – from light pressure to deep interrogation – provides its own information. Alternate working at both superficial and deep levels should be practised, progressively enlarging the examined area, in order to become aware of the varieties in tension between the different levels.

Different specific massage techniques are recognized; each is used for a specific purpose:

1. With the flat of the hands.
2. With the fingertips.
3. With the elbow.
4. Mobilizing massage.
5. To relieve inflammation and prevent adhesions.
6. To restore posture (of the flexor tendons).
7. Drainage massage.
8. Vibratory massage on points of tension.
9. Massage on specific acupuncture points.
10. Reflex massage to stretch the skin, using the fingertips.
11. Deep transverse massage.

[1] J. de Goldfiem. *Physiologie de cheval*. La peau et les phanères, 1er fascicule, Mars 1971.

(1) With the flat of the hands

This light preparatory massage (see photo 1) involves gentle pressure administered with the palms and flattened fingers. It serves as an introduction for the masseur, who is able to take an initial 'reading' of the zones of tension. It also serves to calm the initial anxiety of the horse at being touched.

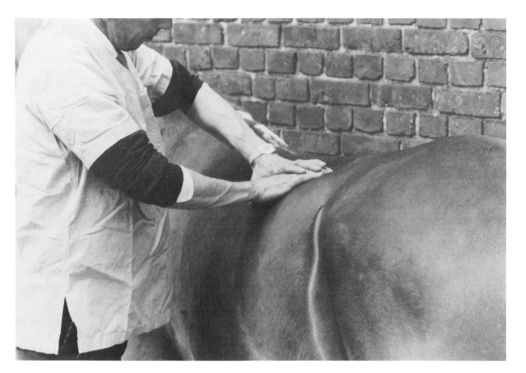

Photo 1 Massage with the flat of the hands.

(2) With the fingertips

The hands are placed against each other (photo 2), with the fingertips joined together to provide more power and precision.

(3) With the elbow

The elbow is completely flexed as shown in photo 3. It is important that the flat part – the triangle formed by the humeral condyle and olecranon – is used rather than the point itself. This method has a powerful action, and should be practised with moderation and care. The back should not be seen to cave in or shrink away. The elbow is placed in the gaps between and around the vertebrae after stretching the hock towards the croup, working in and out with oblique movements. To treat problems in the lumbar region, the technique is performed using circular movements at the ilio-lumbar intersection on the mid gluteal muscle.

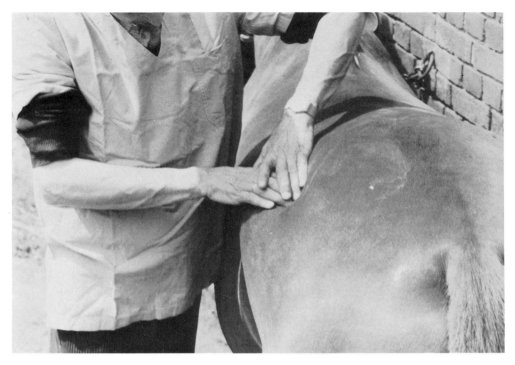

Photo 2 Massage with the fingertips.

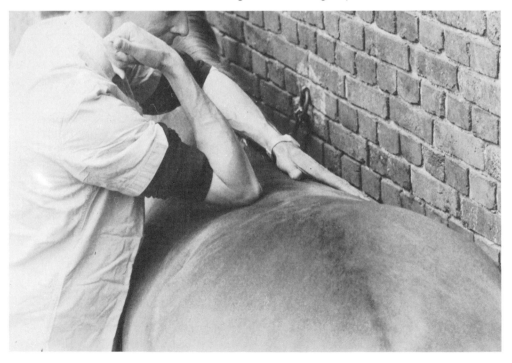

Photo 3 Massage with the elbow.

As a general rule, it is advisable to begin with the flat of the hands, then move on to working with the fingertips, in order to treat the initial spasms. Massage with the elbow is particularly useful for treating the gluteal muscles and insertions of the sacro-iliac muscles.

(4) Mobilizing massage

This technique, illustrated in photo 4, is used to loosen up a muscle (e.g. the brachiocephalic and caudal femoral muscles). It takes the form of petrissage, a firm kneading movement using the palms of both hands; the body of the muscle is moved back and forth by using postural movements.

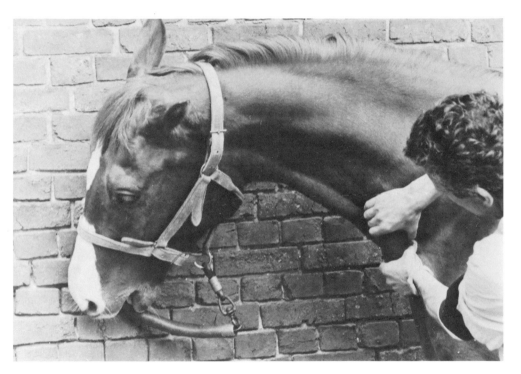

Photo 4 Mobilizing massage (petrissage).

(5) To relieve inflammation and prevent adhesions

As illustrated in photo 5, this technique involves rolling and lifting a fold of skin between the hands. It is very effective in preventing adhesions in the areas where there is a build-up of fibrous scar tissue. It can also be applied to the areas around the vertebral spinous processes. The technique also separates the various layers of skin where the products of inflammation lodge during cellulitis. This powerful massage can, however, be painful, so it should be practised slowly and carefully.

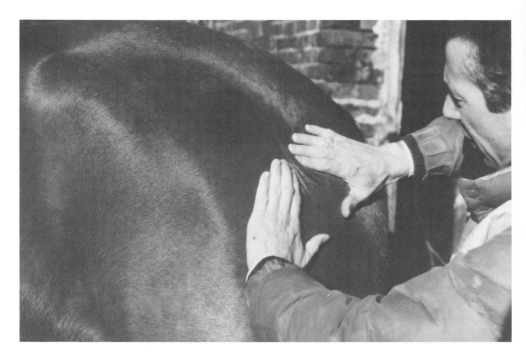

Photo 5 Massage for removing adhesions and separating muscle fibres.

(6) To restore posture (of the flexor tendons)

The same technique is used as in (4), but is applied to the tendons. As shown in photos 6 and 7, the area to be treated is supported and worked from both sides by the thumb and fingers. The massage takes the form of a series of movements in the spaces surrounding the tendon, which stretch and reposition it at the same time. The separate tendinous and ligamentary levels are identified and worked on individually. Oedomatous infiltrate is taken into account.

In a single massage session one should alternate at regular intervals between this technique and the drainage technique discussed in the next section. As always, progressive care and gentleness are the watchwords. Provided that it is respects the condition of the tissues, massage will always be beneficial. The application of pressure to help correct posture steadily increases over the course of the session, and should never be traumatic.

Simple light massage will suffice if an inflammatory area which has not stabilised (e.g. due to serious and recent tendinitis) is suspected. In such circumstances, the appropriate action is several days of lymphatic drainage without direct action on the tendon itself.

(7) Drainage massage

In order to reabsorb lympho-haemorrhagic discharge (e.g. from a swollen limb or torn muscle), one should start with light massage movements, with hands flat and forming a bracelet around the affected limb, sliding to another part of the body while maintaining pressure. Begin in

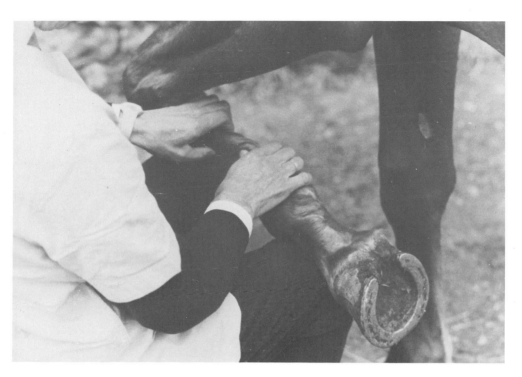

Photo 6 Massage to restore posture: placing under tension.

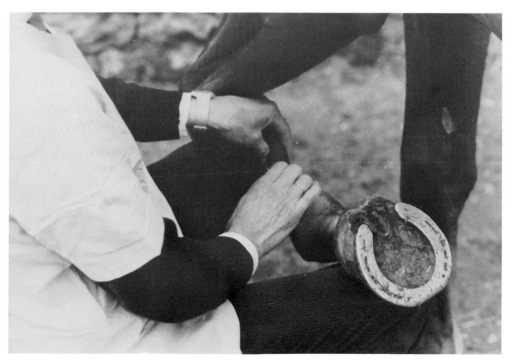

Photo 7 Massage to restore posture: relaxing.

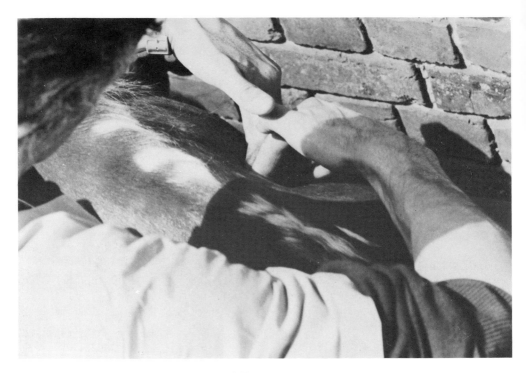

Photo 8 Vibratory massage.

an area distal to that affected, moving from the knee towards the elbow, and from the pastern towards the knee, 5 to 10 minutes in each area, massaging vigorously and alternating the movements. The massage should be followed by a very light, gentle shower, little more than a dribble, applied to the whole limb for 15 minutes. A very thick semi-compressed bandage wound around the whole leg complements the therapy. It should be checked and reapplied every 24 hours, following the daily massage.

Deep massage is not advised for cases of phlebitis as it can encourage dissemination and embolism.

(8) Vibratory massage on points of tension

The fingertips are placed on the points of tension (photos 8 and 9). This technique is for the treatment of muscle spasms. Pressure is applied to the acupuncture points very close to the affected area.

(9) Massage on specific acupuncture points

This massage is performed with two fingers or the thumb on the acupuncture points (photo 10). The movements are small, and alternately superficial and deep; 5 minutes should be spent on each point.

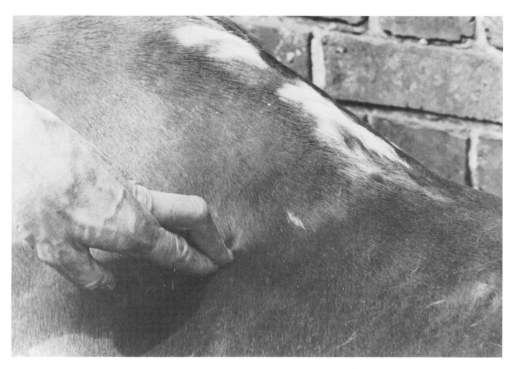

Photo 9 Vibratory massage.

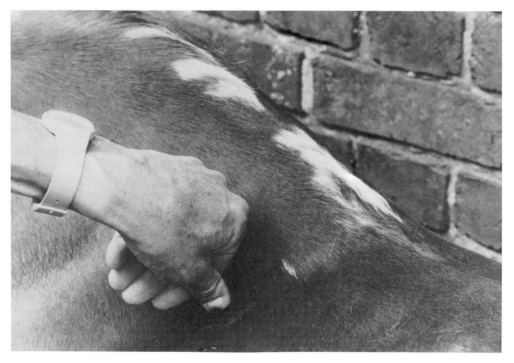

Photo 10 Massage of acupuncture points.

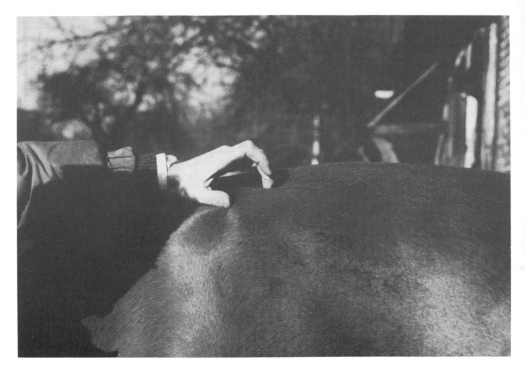

Photo 11 Stretching the skin.

(10) Reflex massage to stretch the skin, using the fingertips

This technique involves the use of the middle finger, which is semi-flexed and assisted by the fourth and fifth fingers to provide additional strength and support (photo 11). It can also be practised counter to the direction of the hair. Following the rules prescribing treatment by area (see Chapter 4, page 148) press deeply, tracing a line on the skin. The skin reacts by swelling slightly along the traced line, as the pressure releases histamine, dilating the blood vessels.

(11) Deep transverse massage (DTM)

DTM is used to treat the ligaments, tendons and muscle insertions in the aponeuroses (photo 12). It is performed transverse to the fibres, with movements which are initially rapid and superficial, and then slower and deeper. One should work with the middle and ring fingers joined together or with the thumb. The deeper massage movements should begin gently to minimize possible trauma, and alternated with the less penetrating ones. The session should last 10 minutes, switching between deep and superficial every 30 seconds. The fingers should remain in constant contact with the skin throughout.

DTM should be used with care on the hocks, where there is a neuro-vascular bundle on the anterior internal face. One should be familiar with the position of the collateral ligaments in order to avoid pressing into the veins on the joints. This very effective massage must be practised with care.

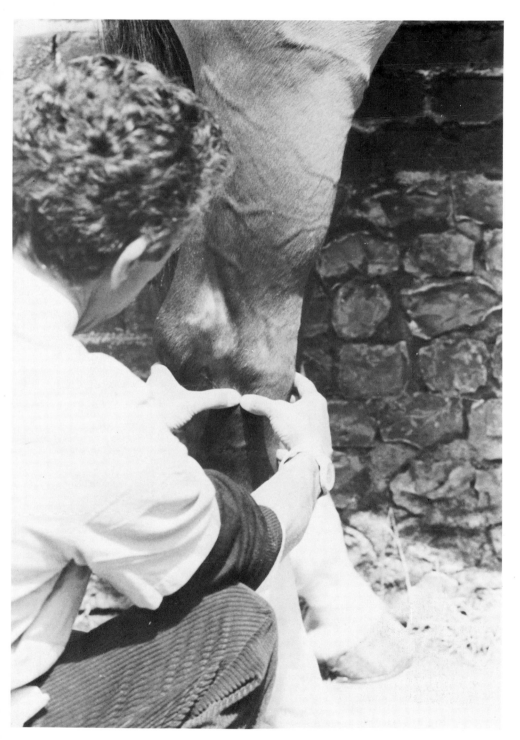

Photo 12 Deep transverse massage.

2. PHYSIOTHERAPY

2.1 ELECTROTHERAPY

(a) Types of current
Three types of current are used: low, medium and high frequency.

1. LOW FREQUENCY CURRENTS
These consist of simple unmodified pulses which can be unmodulated, such as galvanic (iontophoresis, see below), faradic and sinusoidal currents (which can also be combined with galvanic currents). The frequency range is between 0 and 1500 Hertz (cycles per second). Frequency, amplitude and duration can all be modulated; there are a great number of possible combinations, although some have particular physiological properties and are selected for this reason. The therapeutic effects include vasodilatation, resorption of oedema, sedation and excito-motor stimulation.

2. MEDIUM FREQUENCY CURRENTS
The frequency range is between 3 and 10 kHz. For medical purposes an unmodified pulse of the sinusoidal type is used. Medium frequency currents are particularly useful in interferential therapy (photo 13). The therapeutic effects include raising of temperature and vasodilatation.

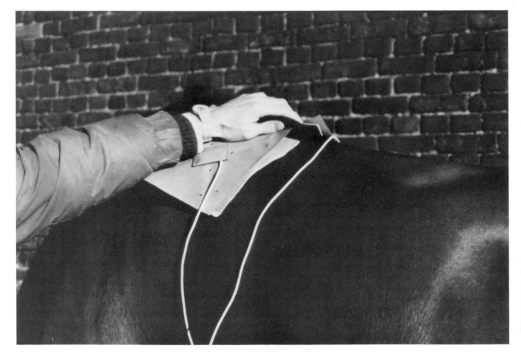

Photo 13 Interferential therapy using medium frequency currents.

3. HIGH FREQUENCY CURRENTS
These are alternating currents with a frequency of 100 kHz and above and cause electromagnetic (hertzian) waves. They have an extended spectrum, but only certain frequencies are used medically. The therapeutic effects include raising of temperature and vasodilatation. They are also used to remove tissue and have surgical applications.

(b) Iontophoresis
1. INDICATIONS
Pain in the joints, sprains, pathologies of the ligament and tendon.

2. THERAPEUTIC EFFECTS
Vasodilatation, resorption of oedema, transport of medically useful ions, sedative effect.

3. SOLUTIONS
Frequently used in electrotherapy include:
- 2% calcium chloride applied to the cathode (tendinitis, sprains);
- 1% potassium iodide applied to the anode (tendinitis, lacerations, oedema);
- 2% sodium salycilate applied to the anode (tendinitis, inflammation).

4. TECHNIQUE (photos 14, 15)
The length of treatment should be 30 minutes.

The cathode is placed facing the most sensitive area, with the anode directly opposite. When treating a limb, the electrodes are held in place using a support bandage placed transversally around the treatment area so that they remain damp. In order to treat a muscle the electrodes are positioned longitudinally, a minimum of 5 cm apart, and fixed in position using elastoplast. Long wires are required in order to cope with movement from the horse, although this should not occur often if the intensity of the current is increased gradually. The range of amperage used should be between 15 and 25 milliamps. While clipping the treatment area is recommended, it is important that it should not be shaved, as this can cause the formation of small scars; these can retard the healing process and cause burns. The skin should also be unbroken and have no scar tissue.

For regions of the body other than the limbs the electrodes are positioned longitudinally rather than transversally, with the cathode placed on the most painful area. To keep the electrode sponges clean, a layer of sopalin should be interposed between them and the skin. The sponges should be cleaned and rinsed after use; prior to application they should be rinsed again and squeezed to remove excess water.

2.2 ULTRASOUND

(a) Therapeutic benefits
Ultrasound provides the following therapeutic benefits:

1. Rise in temperature – the waves excite the molecules in the tissues.
2. Increased permeability of membranes, helping to remove traumatic exudate.
3. Breakdown of the fibres in scar tissue.
4. Analgesia, by reducing the speed of conductivity in the nerves.

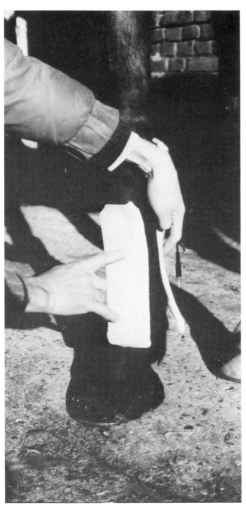

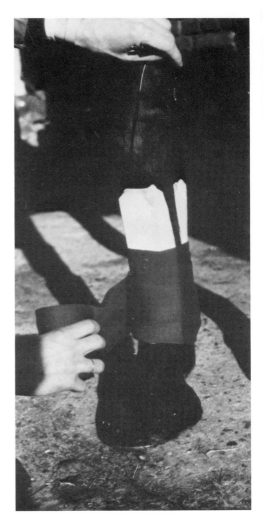

Photo 14 Iontophoresis.

Photo 15 Iontophoresis.

Ultrasound is particularly effective when used together with iontophoresis to treat tenosynovitis, ligamentitis, general ligamentary pain, sprains, joint lesions and lacerations. When applied to the area around the spinous processes, it is also useful for the treatment of spinal problems such as lumbago and inter-spinous ligamentitis.

(b) Technique (photo 16)
Gel should be spread thickly and evenly on the area between the treatment head and the skin to assist penetration; water can also be used. Intensity should be moderated to avoid causing pain and the attendant risk of cavitation. Ultrasound should also not be used within 5 days following an intra-muscular haematoma.

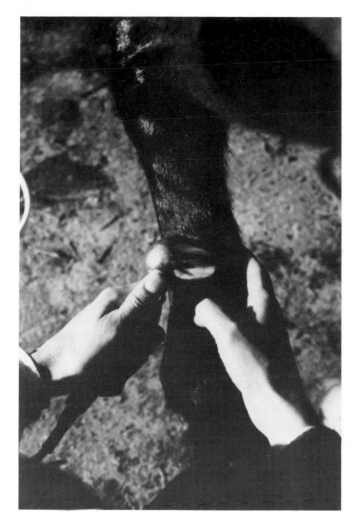

Photo 16 Ultrasound.

For shallow lesions in tendons or ligaments, treatment should be continuous, with an intensity of between 20 and 35 watts, and last 12 minutes – 6 minutes on each side. Using small movements, the treatment head is passed slowly back and forth over the affected area. The best conductor of ultrasound is water, and in cases of tendinopathy the affected limb should be placed in a deep tub. However, it is not always easy to persuade a horse to stand with its foot in water for 12 minutes. Gel should be used in such circumstances; it is effective, even though penetration may be reduced by 50%.

For deep lesions (e.g. in the muscles), ultrasound should be applied in the pulsed mode for 12 minutes, with an intensity of between 35 and 40 watts. If the horse is amenable to having its foot immersed, ice cubes should be added to the water in the tub, and the treatment head applied underwater for 12 minutes.

2.3 LOW ENERGY LASER

Lasers have yet to prove their worth in the treatment of musculo-tendinous problems. Reported benefits are still somewhat ephemeral.

(a) Biological effects of low energy laser

Lasers act at the molecular level, with three principal effects:

1. Cellular – stimulation of the ions within intra-cellular and extracellular tissue, with a bio-regulatory effect.
2. Anti-inflammatory – synthesis of prostaglandins.
3. Analgesic – works on the nervous system's gate control.

Useful depth of penetration is up to 30 mm.

(b) Therapeutic applications

The most conclusive results have been obtained in the treatment of scar tissue repair and revascularization. Laser also seems to be effective for treating ligaments and tendons when combined with the classical therapeutic techniques (iontophoresis, ultrasound). Used on its own, it cannot be relied upon to provide significant muscular repair (e.g. treatment of laceration or lumbago).

2.4 THERMAL THERAPY

There are two methods. *Diffusion* includes the use of thermal mud and green clay, and is more effective than *radiation*, which involves the use of infra-red lamps. Infra-red has a minor role in helping to dry the horse or warm its back prior to work.

2.5 HYDROTHERAPY

Complete immersion of the horse provides conditions of weightlessness suitable for re-education, and exercising in water provides cardiovascular benefits. However, it can cause vertebral overextension, and by interrupting the 'bottom' line can also result in fatigue in the cervico-dorsal area. In a number of training centres in the USA buoys are placed around the horse to help prevent this. Another limitation of this method is that it favours muscular development via the osteo-ligamentary and tendinous system; this system, meeting only minimal proprioceptive and biomechanical resistance, has a tendency to become fragile. Hydrotherapy should therefore be followed by work using the SRP technique described in Chapter 1 as soon as possible. An alternative and effective method which does not suffer from these drawbacks is to use a channel where the water rises as high as the girth, and the horse is massaged under water using jets.

2.6 PHYSIOTHERAPEUTIC ADJUVANTS

(a) Ointments

During the initial period of treatment, ointments which are purely anti-inflammatory or used in conjunction with a neutral cream to prevent skin reactions can be applied. When treatment is for maintenance, massage can be dry, except for the treatment of joints and tendons, where a neutral cream with a gentle active ingredient (e.g. aromatherapy) may be used. After massage the area should be cleaned with a solution composed of one litre of water and 3 tablespoons of synthol. Care needs to be taken with very powerful products during perods when hair is being shed in order to prevent skin reaction. The epidermis reacts more strongly due to heightened activity of the dermis at this level.

It should be borne in mind that it is the massage manipulations which produce the primary therapeutic effects; ointments are at best adjuvants, and must be applied sensitively when treating the joints, ligaments and tendons. Since certain ointments irritate the mucous membranes, a collar should be placed on the horse to prevent licking.

(b) Vibrators

These are very rarely utilized in physiotherapy, and their use as a short-cut is proscribed for anyone who takes therapy seriously. There is no finesse of contact, and the therapist is also prevented from gathering information necessary to treat the patient which can only be provided by touch.

Table 1 Principal medical substances suitable for iontophoresis (from La Galvanotherapie by J. Dumoulin and G. de Bisschop)

Product	Solution	Polarity	Actions	Indications
Adrenalin	2%	+	vasoconstriction	problems with peripheral circulation circulation
Alphachymotrypsin	1%	+	anti-oedomatous	anti-inflammatory contusions, sprains
Cocaine	1% in an alcoholic solution	+	local anaethesia	neuralgia of the trigeminal nerve, shingles
Mepivacaine hydrochloride (Intra-epicaine)	2% w/v in an isotonic solution	seek veterinary advice	local anaesthesia	neuralgia of the trigeminal nerve, shingles
Bichlorhydrate of histamine	0.2%	+	counter-irritant, vasodilatation	rheumatism, joint pain, spasms
Calcium chloride	1%	+	sedative	dysfunction of the sympathetic nervous system, hemiplegia, post- traumatic pain, osteoporosis
Sodium chloride	2%	–	fibrolytic	fibrous scars, keloids
Zinc chloride or sulfate	1%	+	antiseptic	disinfection of the mucous membranes
Potassium citrate	1%	–	anti-inflammatory	rheumatism of the small joints
Gallamine triethiodide (Flaxedil)	4%	amphoteric	removes contractions	contractions, Parkinson's disease
Hyaluronidase	150 units (prepared immediately prior to application)	+	resolvent	chronic lymphoedema, thrombophlebitis, lymphangitis
Potassium iodide	1%	–	vascular, anti-arthritic, fibrolytic	arthritis, arthrosis, moderate pain, adherent scar tissue, keloids
Aconitine nitrate	0.25%	+	analgesic	intense neuralgia
Silver nitrate	29%	+	anti-inflammatory	rheumatic pain in the small joints
Phosphate of epinephrine	1%	+	vasoconstriction	asthma
Corticosteroids Hydrocortisone, succinate of prednisolone	1% 1%	+ –	anti-inflammatory	rheumatism, gout
Sodium salicylate	1%	–	decongestive, analgesic	periphlebitis, acute rheumatism in the joints, myalgia
Copper sulfate	2%	+	antiseptic, fungicide	mycosis, folliculitis
Magnesium sulfate or chloride	25%	+	destructive	common warts
Thiomucase	in solution or as an ointment	–	resolvent	cellulite, lymphoedema, surgical oedemas

Table 2 Indications for the therapeutic application of electrotherapy

Continuous current
- *Thermal elevation, vasodilatation*: of minor importance
- *Polarization of membranes:* very important, with the following effects:
  electroendosmosis (action against oedema)
  sedative action directly applied to nerve endings
  iontophoresis (mobilization of substances)
- *Transport of ions*: very important, quasi-specific, activating medicinal ions including:
  Ca^{++} (sedative)
  I^- (removes hardened tissue)
  Salicylate$^-$ (anti-inflammatory)
  Curararization (stops contractions)
  Histamine (Counter-irritant)
- *Destruction of tissue*: negative electrolysis, aesthetic dermatological applications

Low frequency current
- *Thermal elevation and vasodilatation*: of minor importance
- *Polarization of membranes*: less important than with continuous current, although it has a very important analgesic action. It can be modulated to prevent habituation
- *Transport of ions*: possible if the current is unidirectional
- *Excitomotor action*: this has diagnostic (stimulation/detection) applications and can be used therapeutically on both healthy and diseased tissues

Medium frequency current
- *Thermal elevation and vasodilatation*: more important than continuous and low frequency currents, but less than high frequency
- *Polarization of membranes*: moderate, with a weak sedative action
- *Transport of ions*: not used
- *Excitomotor action*: powerful, tetanizes healthy fibres; modulation and interferential therapy possible, allowing treatment of specific fibres and pulsed tetanization

High frequency current
- *Thermal elevation and vasodilatation*: very important, with nutritive trophic effects
- *Polarization of membranes and transport of ions*: not used
- *Excitomotor action*: none
- *Destruction of tissue*: important, with surgical applications such as coagulation, cutting of tissue and fulguration

Table 3 Ionic solutes for use in electrotherapy

Ions

- Ca^{++}

Salt used:	$CaCl_2$
Concentration:	1%
Polarity:	+

- I^-

Salt used:	KI
Concentration:	1%
Polarity:	-

- Salicylate⁻

Salt used:	Sodium salicylate
Concentration:	3%
Polarity:	+/-

- Mg^{++}

Salts used:	$MgSO_4$
	$MgCl_2$
Concentrations:	2%, 5%, 10%, 20%
	$MgBr_2$
Concentration:	1%, 2%
Polarity:	+

- Li^+

Salt used:	Lithium salicylate
Concentration:	1%
Polarity:	+

- Zn^{++}

Salts used:	$ZnCl_2$
	$ZnSO_4$
Concentration:	1%
Polarity:	+

- Cu^{++}

Salt used:	$CuSO_4$
Concentration:	2 parts per thousand
Polarity:	+

- Citrate⁻

Salt used:	Potassium citrate
Concentration:	1%
Polarity:	-

- Anaesthetics

Salt used:	Mepivacaine hydrochloride (Intra-epicaine)
Concentration:	2% w/v in an isotonic solution
Polarity:	seek veterinary advice

- Vasoconstrictors

Substance used:	Adrenaline
Concentration:	2 parts per thousand
Polarity:	+

- Anti-contractors

Substance used:	Gallamine triethiodide (Flaxedil)
Concentration:	80 mg per litre
Polarity:	+

- Enzymatics

Substance used:	Mucopoly-saccharidase
Concentration:	10 000 TRU per litre (1 bottle of Thiomucase per 10 ml of solution)

- Aconitine

Salt used:	Aconitine nitrate
Concentration:	0.25 parts per thousand
Polarity:	+

- Histamine

Salt used:	Histamine bichlorhydrate
Concentration:	0.20 parts per thousand
Polarity:	+

3 Physiotherapy of Simple Lesions

This chapter describes the lesions which most commonly affect the joints, tendons and muscles, and prescribes the appropriate therapeutic treatment.

1. TREATMENT OF JOINTS

1.1 AETIOLOGY

The origin of the painful lesion can be either traumatic or rheumatic:

1. *Traumatic*. This may be the product of an accident or fall involving sprain. Lesions are graded according to severity, ranging from a simple stretch to laceration of the capsule or ligament;
2. *Rheumatic*. This may be due to congenital or secondary causes, such as poor shoeing and maltreatment. Repeated mini-traumas of the joints, such as those experienced by a young horse being forced to work too hard too early, for example on hard ground with repeated landings, can cause damage to growing bones and cartilages (see pages 99–100). Predisposing causes include nutrition which is deficient in some way; either it is not balanced (e.g. overintake of calcium phosphate due to excessive hay consumption by a young horse) or it is lacking in trace minerals.

1.2 CLINICAL SIGNS

These include chronicity, lameness on hard ground and a positive response to being flexed.

1.3 THERAPY

(a) To treat trauma
1. CRUSHED ICE-PACKS
Wrapped within cloth so that they do not contact the skin directly, these should be applied twice a day, for 45 minutes. At night, warm anti-inflammatory packs should be administered; after removal in the morning, the area should be showered lightly for 20 minutes.

2. MASSAGE
Once a day, as follows:

1. Apply the ointment round the whole joint, working it in against the lay of the hair to achieve maximum contact with the skin.

2. Massage the hollows around the joint; situated within the folds of skin they are more easy to see if the limb is flexed. With deep movements, work the thumb back and forth across these hollows, transversal to the periarticular fibres in the ligaments for 10 minutes. This is the DTM technique mentioned on page 112, which has proved particularly effective in human physiotherapy.
3. It is particularly important not to massage the vascular areas around the joints. When treating the *knee*, this includes the areas behind and inside the joint; when treating the *hock*, the areas in front, where major vessels can be easily felt.
4. Massage prior to walking the horse or before a re-education session.
5. Flex the treated limb for several minutes while working deeply around the tendons and ligaments. Once the limb is held in position, the opportunity should be taken to gently flex and extend the joint.

3. PHYSIOTHERAPY

If electrotherapeutic equipment is available, good results can be obtained by applying iontophoresis for 30 minutes. The solutions applied to the electrodes are 2% potassium iodide (-), 2% sodium salicylate (-) and 2% calcium chloride (+). For sprains of the fetlock joint, ultrasound may be applied for 12 minutes, at 25 to 30 watts.

(b) To treat rheumatism

In many cases, orthopaedic correction is vital. Trimming and shoeing should be discussed with the farrier or vet treating the horse. Extreme care should be taken when operations are aimed at the support or decompression of joint structures. If used excessively, they risk reversing the zones of tension and support and can end up damaging the joint.

1. PHYSIOTHERAPY

In contrast to the treatment of trauma, no cold packs should be used. Instead, warm mud packs should be applied around the affected area for 1 hour per day. The tendons which support the joint and the ligaments around it should be massaged. The technique is less deep than that of DTM; ointment should be applied against the lay of the hair, as described above. Iontophoresis, also applied as described above, is beneficial.

2. ACTIVITIES

After the horse leaves its box, re-educative techniques should be used to help mobilize the joints, walking it ten or so times back and forth in straight lines. This should be continued, combining ascents and descents, for 30 to 40 minutes, without working on the lunge, and avoiding ground that is hard or deep. Warming up should be prolonged and slow, without breaking the cadence, at a jogging pace; there should be no rider, and impulsion and engagement should not be encouraged before the joint shows improvement. The rheumatic joint should be subjected to light and progressive work on a daily basis, in accordance with the dictum that there is no rest day for a horse with this condition.

The joint should be worked on firmly but carefully, without unreasonable expectation of a return to optimum performance. During the week the affected horse should be allowed to work at a basic level, and encouraged to give of its best only at competition.

(c) Windgalls and thoroughpins

The cavities within joints (and the areas where they extend) and the synovial membranes can be the source of dilatation due to hyper-secretion of fluid. Most of the time, this is the product of overexertion on terrain that may be too hard or deep. One should be particularly concerned if windgalls or thoroughpins appear on one or more limbs of a young horse, or if they increase in size. Provided the following basic therapeutic rules are followed, most of these benign swellings should regress rapidly.

1. ORTHOPAEDICS
Check the horse's shoes and posture.

2. WORK
This should be on terrain that is level and not deep (and soft, if the horse is recuperating). Elastic bandages, such as those used for varicose veins, should be applied.

3. PHYSIOTHERAPY

1. In the morning, drainage massage before work and gentle cold showers (lasting 15 minutes) after.
2. In the afternoon, electrotherapy, which does not include ultrasound, but should take the form of low frequency current to encourage excito-motor activity and medium frequency current to provide interferential therapy. This should be followed by massage.
3. At night, astringent wet packs should be applied.

Practised 4 to 5 times a week over two weeks this treatment should be sufficient to provide a return to normalcy.

2. TREATMENT OF TENDONS

2.1 SUMMARY OF ANATOMY AND STRUCTURE

(a) Structure
The tendinous bodies are very long, covering the entire distal part of the limbs. Around the joints they move within sheaths which have synovial membranes which lubricate them. Each tendon is also enveloped by a loose connective tissue rich in elastic fibres called the *paratenon*, the role of which is to enhance the sliding action of the tendon around the joint. Where it comes into contact with the surface of the tendon, the paratenon condenses to form a cellular layer, the *epitenon*, which constitutes the surface wall of the tendon; this is connected to the *endotenon*, which separates the sheaths of tendinous fibres within the tendon.

(b) Constituents

The three main constituents of the tendon are:

1. Fibroblasts, which develop into collagenous fibres;
2. Collagenous and elastic fibres, which provide the tendon with its mechanical properties;
3. A substance rich in mucopolysaccharides which maintains the cohesion of the fibre bundles.

The collagenous fibres are arranged in a three-dimensional helical network which is maintained by the elastic fibres and mucopolysaccharides, giving the tendon its visco-elastic properties.

(c) Blood supply

The circulation of blood through the tendon is precarious. In the Horse, the main vessels enter via the paratenon, branching longitudinally and transversally within the epitenon, and supply a very delicate network within the endotenon.

2.2 TENDON PATHOLOGIES: CLINICAL ASPECTS

(a) Symptoms
1. LOSS OF FUNCTION

1. Lameness which is more or less accentuated according to the severity of the lesion and which does not diminish when walking on soft ground.
2. Interruption in the movement of the fetlock.

2. LOCAL SIGNS
Signs of inflammation around or within the tendon include:

1. Oedematous swelling.
2. Area is hot to the touch;
3. Pain when area is pressed or stretched.

Swellings may vary according to the tendon affected:

1. Superficial flexor – caudal or lateral swelling;
2. Deep flexor – lateral swelling.
3. Suspensor ligament in the fetlock – swelling behind the lateral or medial metacarpus.

Radial and carpal adhesions indicate the presence of deeper injuries.

(b) Aetiology
1. PREDISPOSING FACTORS
These may be anatomical/mechanical or physiological.

1.1 Anatomical/mechanical

1. Lack of steadiness in the feet and in the pastern (straight-jointed).
2. Defective cannon and pastern bones which are either too long or too short.
3. Excessive weight in the area around the shoulders and between the fore-limbs.

1.2 Physiological
These are closely involved with the quality of training and a properly balanced diet. The resistance of tendons and ligaments develops during work. Problems with muscular contraction which can result in tendinous lesions are more likely to occur when the horse is fatigued or suffering an imbalance in its diet. Hypotonia can also be a predisposing condition for ligamentary and musculo-tendinous lesions. If the horse finds itself in difficulties, its corrective reactions to maintain balance and ensure its safety may be too slow. Proprioceptive control improves with training, while development of the cardiovascular system helps ensure that there is an adequate flow of blood to the tendons and muscles.

2. DETERMINING FACTORS

These are traumatic in origin. External traumas include a blow from the hoof of another limb, or poorly fitting bandages and leggings. Internal traumas which produce excessive constraints on the tendon can result from a loss of elasticity in the muscles, overextension of the joints, and mini-traumas arising from the shock generated by repeated impact.

For this reason one should be aware that during locomotion the absorption stage means increased work for the fibrous suspensory ligament in the fetlock, as well as the superficial (perforatus) flexor in the digit and its supplementary ligament, and can result in radial adhesions. In the propulsive phase, the pressure is borne by the deep (perforans) flexor tendon of the digit and its accessory ligament, causing adhesions in the carpal area.

3. LESIONS

1. Sections of the tendon require surgical intervention and hospitalization.
2. Dilacerations may take the form of very minor ruptures, which are painful to the touch and cause lameness at the trot. They can also be more serious, for example when they occur in the suspensory ligament in the fetlock.
3. Peritendinitis manifests as superficial inflammation which does not affect the integrity of the cord of the tendon.
4. Tendinopathy can occur at the point where the collagenous fibres are attached to the osteo-cartilaginous areas at the point of insertion.

4. PROGNOSIS

In all cases it is important, when assessing peritendinous formations, to evaluate the extent to which thickening and engorgement indicate damage to the tendon itself. Engorgement of tissue in the paratenon can occur independently of damage to the tendon and generally resolves itself after two to three weeks of treatment. However, if dilaceration of the tendon results in destruction of collagenous fibres and haemorrhaging, surgical intervention is required. In such cases, physiotherapy has a complementary rather than primary role, that of locomotor re-education.

2.3 PHYSIOTHERAPEUTIC TREAMENT

(a) **General principles**

It is important to remember that the treating of symptoms with corticosteroids is not without certain risks. As pain and swellings diminish in intensity it is easy to overlook the underlying lesion and resume training before it has had time to heal properly. Pain is the body's means of preventing either overwork or an overhasty return to work, and should not subside until the tissues and mechanical properties of the tendon have been restored.

In the Horse, the overall functioning of the musculo-tendinous and osteo-articular system is hampered by two main obstacles during locomotor and proprioceptive re-education – the intensity of constraints, and the limitation of re-educative movements. Physiotherapy can, however, play an important role in the process of re-education.

Tendons, like muscles, are affected by cold and humidity, which can reduce their stretchability and make them more vulnerable. All irregularities in gait and other modifications must be examined closely, as they provide a warning of more serious problems. The main objective is to prevent adhesions and tendinous retractions or elongations.

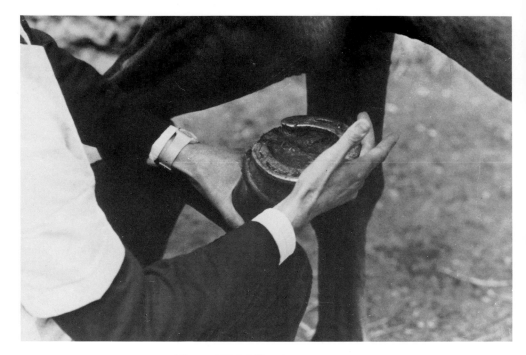

Photo 17 Mobilization massage.

(b) Peritendinitis

There are no indications from the horse's locomotion, but the tendon is hot to the touch. The condition warrants serious attention. There are three stages of treatment: reduction in work, gentle showering of the affected area twice a day and massage according to the following procedure:

1. POSITION

As shown in photos 17 and 18, the therapist is seated on a stool close to the limb to be treated. The limb is flexed at the carpal and the cannon is positioned on the therapist's knee, with the lower part of the leg and foot extending beyond this point. Placing the knee beneath the pastern in this way allows flexion of the fetlock, thus relaxing the flexors. Removing it provokes extension of the joint and puts the flexors under tension. By moving the knee in this way the affected area is placed under a variety of states of tension and relaxation, providing the therapist with much useful information.

2. TECHNIQUE

The tendons are held between the thumbs and fingers of both hands, and, while under tension, massaged using transverse movements.The skin is also worked using a series of gentle detaching movements. The treatment area extends from the pastern-joint to the bend of the carpal. Using this mobilizing technique, each tendon is positioned and worked on separately. The successive tensioning and relaxing created by moving the knee alters the posture in such a way that the paratenon also can be manipulated to drain it or make it more supple. This session, which lasts 15–20 minutes, is followed by a DTM of the collateral ligaments in the area around the fetlock (photo 19). Finally, the tendons are stretched gently by pressing down on the foot 4–5 times for 6 seconds. At no stage should there be a sensitive reaction.

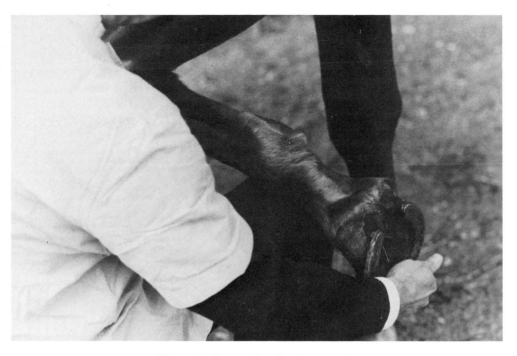

Photo 18 Stretching for 6 seconds.

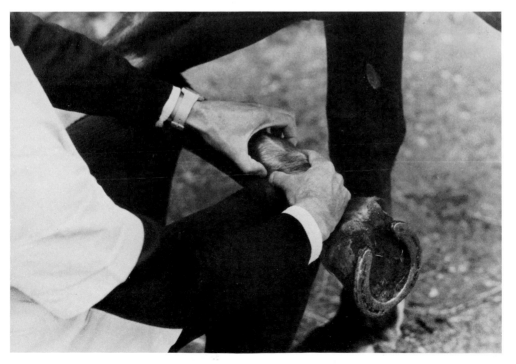

Photo 19 Deep transverse massage of the collateral ligaments.

(c) Dilacerations

However serious or extensive, physiotherapy acts as an adjuvant to more orthodox treatments and can accelerate the return to work.

1. BASES OF TREATMENT

1. Locomotor signs indicate whether work should diminish or cease altogether.
2. Immediate application of iontophoresis is indicated.
3. No treatment by ultrasound within 10 days.

2. SAMPLE TREATMENT FOR A LESION

The treatment period extends from 3 to 5 weeks, bringing together massage, controlled exercise (both walking and at the trot) and electrotherapy. Before the exercise sessions, which should commence as soon as there are no signs of lameness, massage is performed without ointment. Work bandages should never be applied tightly, but positioned with restraint, adjusted properly and held in place by leggings.

Day 1

- *Morning:* massage, 15 min; walk on hard, level ground, 2–3 min; light shower, 15 min.
- *Mid-day:* crushed ice applied around the whole length of the tendon, from the bend of the carpal to just below the fetlock, for 30–40 min. The ice is contained within a bag to prevent direct contact with the skin and to avoid causing a drop in temperature below the recommended 2°C minimum.
- *Early afternoon*: shower, 15 min.
- *Late afternoon*: ice pack, 30 min.
- *Evening:* massage, 15 min; walk, 2–3 min; shower, 15 min.
- *Night:* bandage soaked in a mixture of 2 tablespoons of arnica and 3 of synthol per litre of warm water.

Day 2
As per Day 1.

Day 3

- As per Day 1, but begin the course of electrotherapy prior to the walking session.
- Iontophoresis for 25 min (see photos 14 and 15) with 2% calcium chloride (+), 2% sodium chloride or potassium iodide (-).
- Ultrasound for 12 min at low intensity (25 watts). Apply the head directly using gel, or while the limb is placed in ice water.
- Walking sessions: twice a day for 3 min.

Days 4–7
As above, but extend walking sessions to 5 min on hard ground, 2 min on soft ground.

Days 8–10
As above, but add 2–3 min led at the trot on hard ground.

Days 11–15
As above, but work outside, mounted, 15 min on hard ground. Discontinue the electrotherapy after 10 sessions, although iontophoresis can continue up to 15 sessions if oedema persists. When the horse has regained satisfactory locomotion, massage once in the morning for 15 min, without ointment, prior to work. Maintain the bandages, and shower for 15 min after the session.

3. STRETCHING (photo 20)
As work starts to intensify, around the 4th or 5th week, locomotor re-education can be assisted by stretching sessions. These can be practised either *after* work while the horse is still warm, prior to showering, or *before* work, after 15 min of massage. The initial movements should be manual, and then continue with 3 to 5 very gentle stretchings with the limb placed on a load extender.

Always begin at a point below the painful area. A session should last 3–4 min and consist of a dozen stretching movements alternating with rest phases, both of 10 seconds duration. It is followed by a shower lasting 10–15 min, and application of an ice pack for 30 min.

The techniques when using a load extender vary according to the biomechanical properties of different tendon structures.

1. Placing the tendon of the deep digital flexor and carpal adhesion under tension requires extension of the distal interphalangeal area. This can be produced by placing the horse's foot on a plank 30 cm long, with one end 5 cm above the other to create a slope; one can equally use a longer plank (130–150 cm) which can be raised progressively and precisely to create interphalangeal hyperextensions (Fig. 57). The limb is initially placed on the extender by gripping the withers firmly and moving the horse onto it. The opposing foot is then lifted and the therapist, by controlling the tensioning of the tendon, lifting the fetlock and checking the reactions of the horse, can control the amplitude of the hyperextension.
2. Placing the tendon of the superficial digital flexor and suspensor ligament of the fetlock under tension involves similar procedures, except in this case the heels are raised in order to overextend them and relax the tendon. Short (30 cm) or long (100 cm) planks can be used, and amplitude controlled by monitoring closely the lowering of the fetlock, the state of tension of the tendon and ligament, and the reactions of the horse.

(c) Rehabilitation for performance

It is particularly important to walk the horse as soon as lameness has disappeared; this is to provide the affected area of the tendon with a minimum of mechanical, proprioceptive and vascular support. A few strides at the trot can be introduced. Once the horse is no longer limping at this gait, this training programme of walking interspersed with trotting should be carefully maintained for the following eight days. This period is known as the the 'eight sacred days'.

The exercise is carried out on hard ground. The affected area of the tendon should be massaged before the horse leaves the box. During these sessions, it is preferable to place side reins on the horse, without using them actively, in order to control the horse's reactions during this phase, particularly if the intensity of the work needs to be substantially reduced.

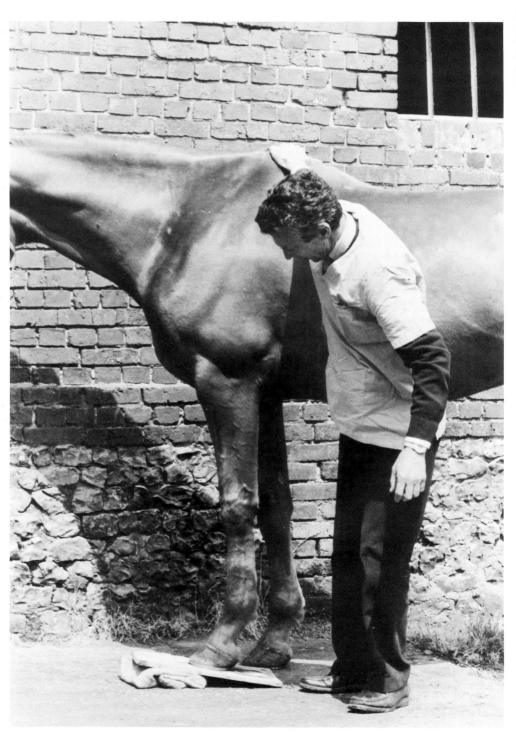

Photo 20 Stretching using the extender.

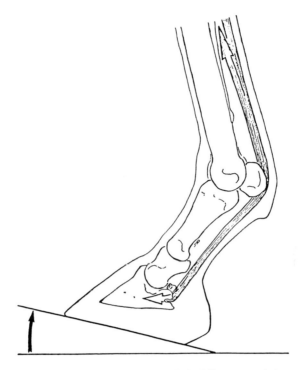

Figure 57 Stretching the tendon of the deep digital flexor and the carpal bar.

3. TREATMENT OF MUSCLES

The painful muscle needs to be analysed quickly; this will assist in planning the re-education programme and avoid inappropriate muscular action during rehabilitation.

3.1 PHYSIOLOGY OF MUSCLE

Muscle is composed of a network of fibrils separated by layers of connective tissue.

1. Myofibrils are richly vascularized, contractile and elastic.
2. Connective tissues are less vascularized, resistant, can be distorted, and lack contractility and elasticity. They can stretch only slightly, unless subjected to tension for a minimum of 6 seconds.

Both components govern aspects of the two principal muscular activities:

1. Contraction, during which the muscle shortens.
2. Stretching, during which the muscle lengthens (particularly in reponse to the contraction of an antagonist)

3.2 JUDGING SYMPTOMS

There are three main ways in which muscular pain manifests:

1. The muscle contracts and shortens (see Fig. 58).
2. The muscle is lengthened as a result of the contraction of its antagonist, or due to an opening caused by leverage (see Fig. 59).
3. 'Active braking'. This consists of eccentric restraint followed by concentric activity. For example, during the cushioning phase in the stride of the rear legs, the femoral quadriceps first 'applies the brakes' to the stifle and then resumes acting concentrically during the propulsive phase.

(a) Functional evaluation

When attempting to assess lameness, a variety of conditions must be looked at, as muscular pain can involve either contraction of the active muscle, or stretching of its anatagonist in response.

For example, if the horse has difficulty in engaging its hind leg (excluding for the time being osteo-articular causes), this may be due either to contraction of the lumbo-gluteal extensors (which are painful to the touch), or to a defect in the functioning of the lumbar or hip flexors. This group can experience pain either during the propulsive phase (concentric contraction) or during the lengthening phase, at the moment when engagement starts to pull on the muscle.

During both of these phases, pain will often be evident in the early stages of movement.

(b) Inspection

Visual examination is important. Both sides of the muscle need to be palpated so that the surface contours and underlying structures can be compared. It is often useful to take a bird's eye view, slightly above the horse, with its head facing you, in order to visualize the symmetry of the muscular reliefs surrounding the vertebral column. A bale of hay can be pressed into service. This technique can reveal a great deal of information; it is particularly useful for assessing vertebral alignment, tension in the trapezius, and the contours of the shoulders.

(c) Palpation: key points and zones of tension

The suffering muscle generates pain in a diffuse way, so it is sometimes difficult to pinpoint the source or key point. This is true of human athletes as well, and can be compared to the way that toothache affects the entire jaw. Manual investigation does not immediately reveal the key point. One must initially deal with the spasm, and two or three sessions of treatment may be necessary before the source can be found. When the tonus of the horse is too high, it obscures musculo-cutaneous messages. In order to create a state of relaxation, the poll should be stroked and the horse spoken to gently; gradually, the true source of the tension will be revealed.

If the horse is reluctant or unable to stand on all four feet, it is very difficult to evaluate the true cause of the spasms; a symmetrical stance is important to obtain a useful map of the zones of tension.

(d) Order of procedures

1. Static examination in the box (visual assessment, palpation, background history).
2. Dynamic examination, while the horse is on the lunge or mounted.
3. In-depth investigation through palpation, again in the box.

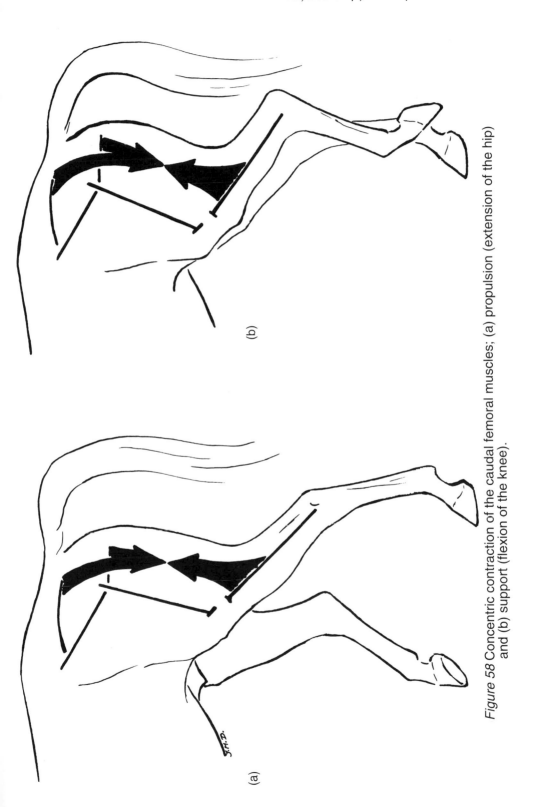

Figure 58 Concentric contraction of the caudal femoral muscles; (a) propulsion (extension of the hip) and (b) support (flexion of the knee).

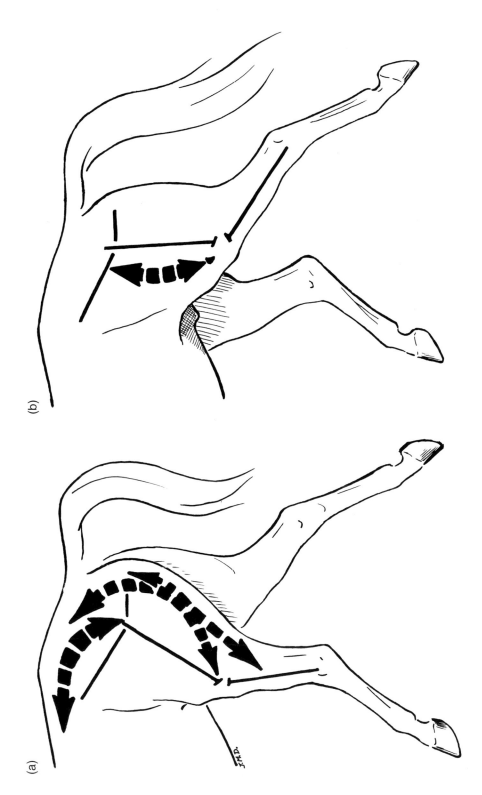

Figure 59 Lengthening of the pelvic and thigh muscles; (a) protraction (lengthening of the gluteal and caudal femoral muscles) and (b) propulsion (lengthening of the rectus femoris and tensor fasciae latae).

This approach differs from classic investigative procedures in that the focus is on the dialogue between the healing, attentive hand and the pain which is being expressed. Hitherto, the dynamic examination together with assessment of the background history has provided the main source of information.

The purpose of palpation is to draw information together from a variety of sources; it summarizes and guides and is a frequent instrument of discovery. The horse's responses are eloquent; it expresses anxiety and surprise, and shrinks away when a painful area is touched. Its gestures and attitudes provide additional confirmation – the limb flexes, the back curves. Communication between therapist and patient starts to take shape and becomes enriched.

3.3 REHABILITATION OF MUSCULAR PERFORMANCE

(a) General approach

One should make every effort to understand the cause of the damage and be aware of the ways in which pain is expressed. The initial task is to find the affected muscle in order to work out the appropriate method of re-education, and establish which movement or dynamic should be retained so that the area around the injury is not deprived of all activity.

For example, the re-educative programme for a laceration of the semispinatus in the left shoulder should proceed as follows:

1. Suspension of work on the right rein in order to avoid stretching.
2. Return to work to be gradual and in a straight line.
3. When working at the trot on the left rein is performed without signs of pain, work on the right rein to be introduced gradually.
4. Muscular movement during the stretching phase of the programme, which involves incurvation of the side opposite the injury, should not be introduced until after scar tissue has formed in order to avoid the risk of new lacerations.

When the site of the lesion has been located accurately and the biomechanics and various roles of the muscle assessed, the therapist can then establish:

1. *Direction* and *amplitude* of movement.
2. *Gait* and *duration* of work.
3. *Load* (with or without rider).

(b) Treatment procedure

1. AVOID STRETCHING THE AREA WHERE THE LESION IS SITUATED

The main rule is to avoid stretching in an area which is inflamed and where scar tissue is forming; work in the re-educative programme should always be designed with this in mind. A particular incurvation is chosen carefully and adhered to until the muscle is healed. Examples of the application of this rule can be seen in the treatment of myalgia of the paravertebral muscles and of the limbs.

1.1 Paravertebral myalgia

The horse is worked at the volte for lesions situated laterally; the painful muscle is situated within the concave area created by the volte to avoid stretching it (Fig. 60). If, for example, the myalgia occurs on the left side of the trapezius or erector spinae, the horse should be worked on the same side for 8 to10 days, until palpation has revealed a clear improvement. Walking

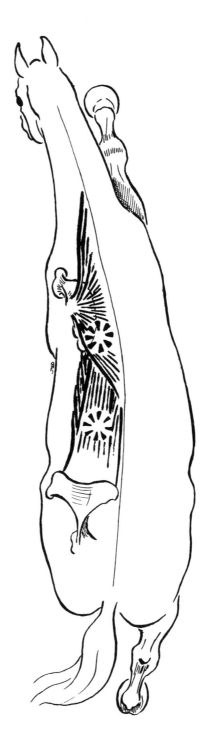

Figure 60 Homolateral incurvation to avoid stretching sites of lesions.

with incurvation on the opposing side is then introduced very gradually. If incurvation shortens the paravertebral muscles causing pain, the horse should be worked in straight lines on the lunge, making the voltes very large.

Ventral flexion in the lumbar region is not sufficiently powerful to induce stretching; it has an additional benefit in that it obstructs the messages of pain originating in the neuro-muscular spindles.

1.2 Myalgia in the limbs

Restraint is placed on the engagement of the propulsive muscles in the posterior of the thigh and croup and on the amplitude of movement of the retractor muscles in the forelimb. Restricting the musculo-articular dynamic in this way helps control movements which would otherwise lengthen muscular fibres which need to be allowed time to heal. Much later, the programme of rehabilitation includes stretching, provided that its extent is limited, that the horse's muscles are warmed up, and that it is tolerated. This will help avoid stiffness the following morning.

2. CRITERIA FOR MUSCULAR RE-EDUCATION

2.1 Direction

The activity of the muscle must be controlled by working the horse with incurvation on the same side as the injury, restraining its movements to avoid significant lengthening of the muscle fibres.

2.2 Amplitude

This should be reduced to the point that it almost prevents impulsion, so that the horse is jogging, with a noticeably choppy trot. When the horse is no longer feeling discomfort, it is allowed to extend the movement working with the volte on the affected side. It is then walked in a straight line and made to change direction, with the initial steps again at walking speed.

2.3 Duration

Each day extend the period of work by 5 to 10 minutes.

2.4 With or without rider

For muscular problems in the area around the shoulder and arm and in the dorsal thoracic region, rehabilitation should proceed without the weight of the rider until the signs of inflammation – pain, heat and contraction – have subsided. With problems in the lumbo-gluteal area, the horse may be ridden sooner at a slow and controlled walking speed.

For other problems in the shoulder/arm area the rider should not place his full weight in the saddle and position it further back than usual, bringing the chest area up and raising the front of the horse. Conversely, for problems of the back and hindquarters, the rider should stand in the stirrups and carefully balance himself well forward in order to free up the dorso-lumbar area.

2.5 Organization of the return to work

This stage should commence when the horse is no longer exhibiting signs of lameness or sensitivity. Work is always preceded by a 15 min massage. The horse is worked on the affected side for 15 min on the lunge, and then for a further 15 min on the other rein. For lesions which occur at the junction between tendon and muscle, work (while mounted) is followed by shower or application of ice packs for 15 min, and a half-hour later, massage for 15 min.

For muscular problems involving laceration, massage is applied immediately to the affected area. Movements are gentle, anti-spasmodic and circular, performed with the flat of the hand along the whole of the muscle. Medium frequency (interferential) electrotherapy or ultrasound help complete the process of forming scar tissue. These treatments are applied for 8 to 10 days.

3.4 SPECIAL THERAPEUTIC TECHNIQUES

Treatment of different types of muscular lesion.

(a) Contusion

Lesions caused by direct impact, or which occur as a result of violent effort, accompanied by intramuscular haematoma. Whatever the degree of seriousness, the treatment is the same:

1. Rest in the box.
2. Application of ice-pack once a day (within a bag so that temperature of the skin does not fall below 2 to 4°C); warm anti-inflammatory packs at night.
3. Very gentle showers, alternately hot and cold, 2 to 3 times a day for 10 to 15 min.
4. Lymphatic drainage massage in the immediate area without touching the lesion itself.
5. If no signs of lameness at the beginning of the 3rd day following the injury, the horse can be led at the walk.
6. Ultrasound, either pulsed or continuous, max. 30 watts, at the beginning of the 6th day.
7. Iontophoresis.

1. REHABILITATION

1. Establish which side the lesion is situated on; the re-educative programme involves incurvation on the same side, particularly when the paravertebral muscles are affected. Intramuscular haematoma must not be subjected to pressure as there is a risk of bleeding.
2. No corticosteroids should be given as there is a risk of bleeding, and no ultrasound treatment before the 6th day.
3. Excitomotor electrotherapy should start on the 6th day. This can be accompanied by 2 to 3 sessions of mesotherapy, which involves the use of tiny needles. The combination of the two is beneficial.

(b) Contraction, lengthening

If the horse is not allowed to rest from sporting activity, this can be the precursor to laceration. Work should be slow and relaxing for 2 weeks and accompanied by the following therapeutic programme:

1. Application of a mud pack for 30 min, once a day.
2. Massage of the point of tension, near to the source of pain.
3. Ultrasound, excitomotor electrotherapy.
4. Avoidance of cold.
5. Work with the appropriate incurvation to avoid causing pain, until signs of muscular contraction have ceased.
6. If sensitivity is no longer evident, work should proceed in a straight line, then with the opposing incurvation.

(c) Muscular laceration

Rest is strictly prescribed to keep haematoma to a minimum. Palpation is the best means of detecting changes in the contours of muscles which reveal the presence of intramuscular fluid. Visible protuberances, it goes without saying, are evidence of a more serious injury.

Laceration requires a minimum of one month of careful treatment. If that care, and rigorous training, are not forthcoming, lameness can be expected to last for several months. A typical example is lameness in the shoulder, which is notoriously long-lived. Diagnosis is often difficult, and anti-inflammatory treatments mask the pain momentarily, leading to premature resumption of work thus causing new lesions. Treatment is the same as for contusion with intramuscular haematoma.

1. Absolute rest so that the haematoma is reduced to the minimum, as bleeding can continue for several days.
2. For lacerations situated in the shoulder area, massage can reveal the site of the lesion very precisely. Daily massage provides the greatest source of information on problems in the shoulder.

It is worth relating a case-history at this point.

A horse became lame in the left shoulder after panicking in a van, with a forced incurvation on its left side. The first session was able to uncover nothing more than a considerably swollen latissimus dorsi muscle. After three massages, however, the sites of the lesion were precisely located. The pain in the thoracic trapezius, very intense at the outset of treatment, was rapidly relieved. The latissimus dorsi remained swollen and painful but one could feel the laceration in the infraspinatus. Without this daily, deep probing, the nature of the lesions would not have been revealed and the appropriate treatment would not have been so precise.

Incurvation on the side of the injury, thus shortening the muscle fibres, is also indispensable for treating laceration during the phase of rehabilitation. Working the horse when mounted is proscribed until there is confirmation of progress and an absence of lameness.

1. RE-EDUCATION IN THE BOX

At the beginning of the 6th day, for injuries to the neck and shoulder area, movements of the neck can be encouraged through games. The horse, confined to its box, should find them diverting. For example, a balloon can be attached to a piece of string and suspended next to the horse's head, or held in place by 2 or 3 thicker pieces of twine 80 cm in length which are tied to the ground. The horse will move its neck and shoulders trying to make the pieces of twine move or play with the balloon.

4 Treatment by Area

1. NECK AND POLL

In the Horse, the neck section is most flexible part of the vertebral column. There are three main potential sources of problems:

1. Congenital structural defects, including inversion.
2. Maltreatment. As described in Chapter 3 (see page 91), the spine, of which the neck is a part, acts as an emotional filter; one often finds that problems in this area, such as inappropriate muscular development, spasms and contractions, are the product of tensions caused by the rider or his methods of work.
3. Trauma, including all lesions caused by accidents, such as falls, etc.

Compared with the dorso-lumbar bridge, which has to bear the weight and movements of the rider, there are fewer directly biomechanical reasons for the neck to be problematic. However, situated as it is, directly in front of the rider, it presents an powerful means of control; all too often, use of this control acts as a brake on the horse's locomotion, engendering defensive tensions in the paravertebral area which have an effect on overall biomechanical performance. Most of the major commentators, including Steinbrecht, have underlined the danger of forcing the developing young horse to raise its head prematurely, which can cause inward distortion of the cervical spine.

1.1 GLOBAL APPROACH

(a) Locating problem areas (Fig. 61)
When locating specific points of tension, it should be borne in mind that problems anywhere along the vertebral column can have repercussions in the neck and poll. Behaviour patterns well known to riders include:

1. Resistance to flexions of the head and poll.
2. Uncertain or jarring movements – the horse cannot 'settle down'.
3. Resistance to control, defensive movements.
4. Tightening of the trapezius and rhomboid muscles in the shoulders, limiting extension.
5. Resistance to or refusal to allow incurvation.

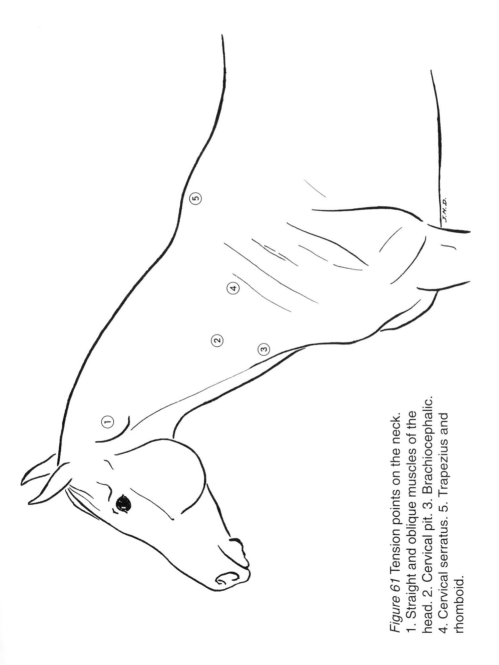

Figure 61 Tension points on the neck.
1. Straight and oblique muscles of the head. 2. Cervical pit. 3. Brachiocephalic. 4. Cervical serratus. 5. Trapezius and rhomboid.

(b)Treatment

When the point of tension – most often due to muscular problems – has been identified by palpation, a number of massage and other physiotherapeutic techniques can be used (photos 21, 22 and 23). The treatment for laceration is described on pages 130–131. Contractions and myalgias, which can be either rheumatic or traumatic in origin, are treated once a day prior to work, as follows:

1. Ultrasound – 12 min, in a wide arc around the affected area; 25–30 watts if continuous, 35–40 watts if pulsed.
2. Massage – 15–20 min; one should work with gentle transverse movements, focusing on the affected muscle, progressively deeper so that it can be felt moving under the fingers, but without eliciting a painful response.
3. Medium frequency (interferential) electrotherapy – 15 min, moving from one side of the neck to the other, again without eliciting a painful response.
4. Low frequency electrotherapy involving transcutaneous stimulation of the nerves – 10 min at 5 Hz then 10 min at 80 Hz. This technique must not be used higher up the neck as it can frighten the horse. Changes in intensity must also be introduced very gradually for the same reason.

1.2 PRINCIPAL POTENTIAL PROBLEM AREAS

(a) Poll and mid-neck (areas 1 and 2)

1. SYMPTOMS
The horse (a) resists or has difficulty in laterally flexing its head; (b) shakes its head; (c) does not free the bit – this is associated with dorso-lumbar resistance originating from problems in the nuchal region.

2. TREATMENT
Start in area 1, with gentle tranverse massage of the retro-occipital region for 5-10 min, until the neck relaxes and lowers. The massage is most effective if the horse lowers its poll. Probe deeply with the fingertips using circular movements. Move down towards area 2.

(b) Brachiocephalic (area 3)

1. SYMPTOMS

1. Contractions, which can either be isolated within the muscle itself or connected to problems in the shoulder.
2. Limited protraction of the limb.
3. Knotted shoulders; extension of the shoulder or forearm is limited or painful.

2. TREATMENT
Mobilizing massage of the whole muscle, starting at the lower insertions and working a third of the way along. Combine with petrissage movements (see page 107) for 5 min. Stretch the rear of the leg while rocking the shoulder.

Photo 21 Neck and poll.

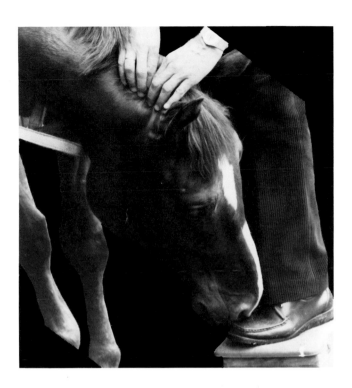

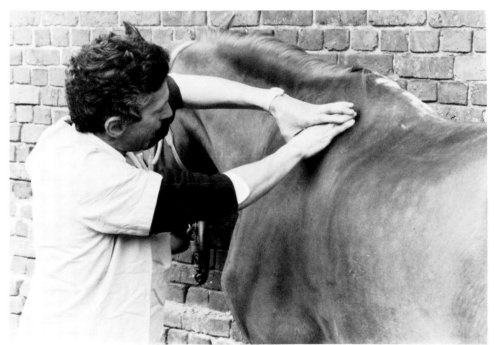

Photo 22 Neck and poll.

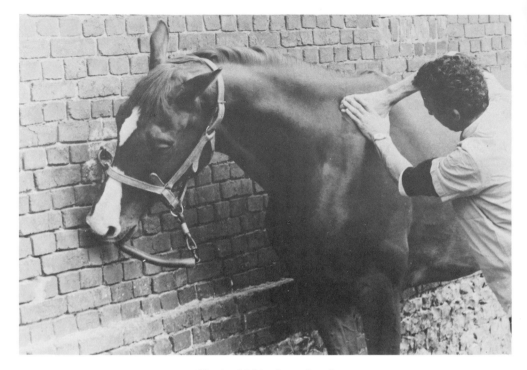

Photo 23 Neck and poll.

(c) Serratus (area 4) and trapezius and rhomboid (area 5)

1. TREATMENT

The practitioner should draw the muzzle towards himself in order to cause incurvation of the neck, and massage area 4 deeply using the fingertips. One hand massages while the other maintains the incurvation. Area 5 is of special interest, as both cervical and dorsolumbar pathologies are treated here. Massage with the flat of the hands and then with the fingertips, following the edge of the scapula and working the fibres transversally. Tension in this area can cause a loss of scapulo-humeral mobility and resistance to flexion and incurvation in the neck.

1.3 COMPLEMENTARY TREATMENT

(a) Massage of the acupuncture points

Fig. 62 indicates the position of line 36, which should be massaged with 10 strokes. Punctiform massage, using the fingertip or with the finger slightly bent, and without eliciting a painful reponse, should be performed for 5 min on points 37, 40, 39 and 7. This should be followed by gentle massage of the retro-occipital area for 5 min.

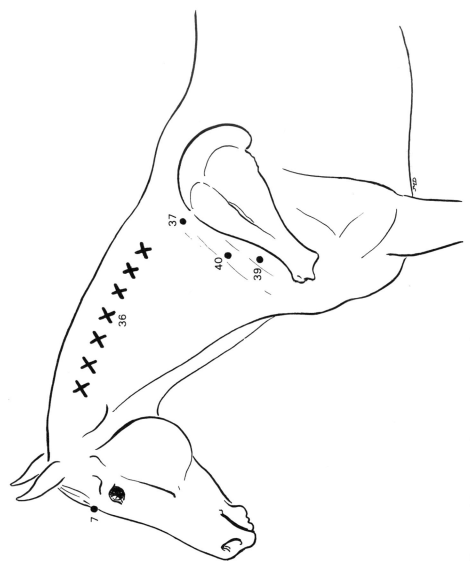

Figure 62 Massage of acupuncture points.

(b) Reflex massage
See Fig. 63.

1. At the anterior edge of the scapula, in front of the subclavius, working from top to bottom, 5 successive strokes which cause linear stretching of the skin.
2. Comma-shaped strokes, approximately 10 cm long, working from the poll towards the scapula. Each stroke should be performed twice.
3. The same strokes, again performed twice, following the path of the brachiocephalic from the upper insertion downwards.

This is then followed by 3 strokes along the anterior edge of the scapula. To conclude the session, face the horse, apply 3 or 4 downward strokes to each side of the neck; start at the sub-occipital region, initially pressing heavily with 2 or 3 fingers, then massaging with the flat of the hands. Repeat.

At this stage it is important to mention the nervous connections between dermatomes (areas of skin supplied with afferent nerve fibres by a single posterior spinal root), myotomes (muscles innervated from a single spinal segment) and certain viscera. Stimulation of a dermatome will trigger a reflex response in the connected myotome and viscera.

1.4 TECHNIQUES OF RE-EDUCATION

(a) In the box

1. Isometric contractions, using a minimum of movement.
2. As described on page 141, a piece of string with balloon attached at head height, or thicker pieces of string, with which the horse can play.

(b) Outside
Resume work with reins to re-establish and stabilize neck movements. The neck should then be lowered, using prudent incurvations; working on both reins helps ensure that the neck is worked equally on either side.

2. THE BACK

2.1 INTRODUCTION TO VERTEBRAL PHYSIOPATHOLOGY

Periarticular and interspinous ligaments are often the source of inflammatory reactions. It is around the anchorage points of the ligaments that the first osteophytic calcifications develop; these signal incipient ligamentitis which is the initial stage of numerous vertebral arthroses.

Within the paravertebral muscles, neuromuscular dysfunction can result in a reflex contraction or cramp – what Antonietti has termed a 'pathological reflex to blockage in function' or PRBF – together with a lack of co-ordination between agonist and antagonist muscles. The blockage is caused by the vertebral column becoming concave as an analgesic defensive measure, with simultaneous reduction of space within the concave side and opening up of a gap on the convex side. Damage to the spinal and sympathetic nerve fibres in the area of the blockage can affect muscular trophism and vascularization.

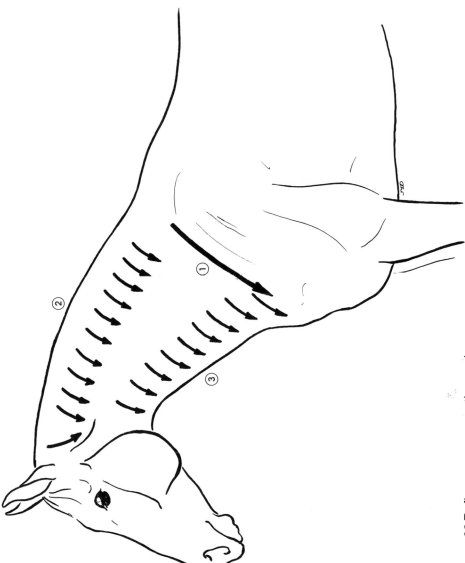

Figure 63 Reflex massage on the neck.

2.2 THE THERAPEUTIC APPROACH

Therapeutic treatment of the spasms affects the dermatomes as much as the corresponding myotomes; the distance from the affected area varies according to the gravity of the lesion.

The sequence of therapeutic treatments (reflex massage) at the cutaneous level is of clear importance. When treating PRBF there should be an initial pre-mobilizing massage and then a mobilizing analgesic massage. Manipulations of the skin, fascia, muscles and tendinous ligaments help calm paravertebral reflexes, which are most often a response to pain in the myo-fascial area. The causes of these reflexes are varied – overwork, terrain which causes neurotony (stretching of a nerve), metabolic problems, the poor preparation and disrupted work patterns affecting the muscular chains.

2.3 PATHOLOGY

Actual vertebral displacement in the horse is rare. The overlapping of the vertebral bodies and articular surfaces limits movement of the thoraco-lumbar spine. The cervical spine, as a result of its greater mobility and exposed position, is more frequently subject to traumas resulting from accidents.

The great majority of vertebral problems involve muscular and ligamentary dysfunction – simple and reflex contractions, supra- and interpinous ligamentary dystrophy, incipient overlapping of the spinous processes (OSP) and consequent periosteal modification (which is detectable using radiology).

In his paper 'Conditions causing thoraco-lumbar pain and dysfunction in horses' Jeffcott concluded that damage in this area is most frequently linked to problems of temperament as well as to poor coordination in very highly-strung horses. He placed particular emphasis on the impact of severe spasms on the performance of the longissimus muscle. When looking at his table on the origins of dysfunction it is interesting to note that out of 825 horses examined, he discovered 269 cases of musculo-ligamentary lesions, 234 cases of OSP, 118 cases of lesions of the sacro-iliac ligament and only 1 case of lumbar vertebral displacement!

These observations should make us consider the importance of musculo-ligamentary symptoms when vertebral problems occur, as well as being the possible cause of those problems. Several conclusions may be drawn from this:

1. Poor direction, inadequate preparation and uncontrolled movements result in recurring muscular tensions (this is statistically verifiable).
2. Calm results in sound movements and agitation in the opposite.
3. The initial stage of OSP, affecting as it does the ligaments and periosteum, shows the importance of work on the thoraco-lumbar area (including the necessity of hyper-extension).

Jeffcott felt that thoraco-lumbar displacement was of minor importance; he considered muscular spasms, which exerted pressure where the muscles crossed over the joints, to be the chief cause of curvature (spastic scoliosis) of the spine. This is supported by observations in human physiotherapy. Tensions in the vertebral joints are frequently eased when the therapist treats spasms resulting neuromuscular activity within the muscles which perform the subtle movements of the spine.

2.4 SYMPTOMS

(a) Seeking out the causes of paravertebral musculo-ligamentary disorders

One begins by pushing with small tension-producing thrusts against the horse's flank, using the movement of the stomach to create light imbalances. Placing the hands far apart on the paravertebral muscles, the therapist can then start to 'read' the behaviour of the layers of muscles and examine the details of the contours and the depth of the different reliefs, both periarticular and fibrous. The gentle waves transmitted to the spine by movements of the therapist's body reveal pathologies in stance which are caused by the cybernetic frame producing support for movement when the horse is over-exerting itself.

The wealth of information thus obtained is rapidly supplemented by therapeutic contact with the healing hand. Massage cannot be understood outside of the context of mobilization, during which the fibres are worked on manually to release tensions in the areas around the fibro-cartilaginous insertions. During the healing dialogue, the therapist releases, channels, listens, and follows the resorption of spasms at various levels and depths within the horse's body.

When treating the lumbar and sacro-iliac region, the therapist positions himself facing the hip or behind the horse. The process of observation continues, with the same oscillations and small movements used again to obtain information both from the surface and from deep within the horse's body.

The muscles of the scapula or hip and all those surrounding the joints must be examined using the same approach. The various massages associated with muscular tensions accomplish a similar purpose and treat the symptoms of spasticity generated by many reflex problems. The normalization of vertebral 'displacement' is frequently nothing more than the resolution of a musculo-ligamentary or cybernetic problem which has been accelerated by massage treating the true cause.

Stiffness will make the whole area rigid; to prevent this occurring, the therapist uses his body and fingers to exert pressure, stretch, laterally flex, and flex and extend the area, using small movements. Muscular cords and points of tension which indicate complex blockages are revealed. Tensions, capsular inclusions and compressions of the cartilage can be maintained by muscular contractions, particularly at the level of the inter-apophyseal joints. As the insertions of the deep muscular chains are involved and increase reflex activity, it is important to break the cycle.

(b) The principal points of tension

These are indicated in Fig. 64.

Zone 1: thoracic and cervical trapezius muscles; on a deeper level, the rhomboideus.

Zone 2: located behind the withers are the anterior anchorages of the extensors of the back. In many cases, the paraventral dorso-lumbar section of the muscular chain can lock and be the source of pain in this area.

Zone 3: a key point for back pain, due to the pressure of the cantle. Investigation should extend as far as the iliocostal muscle.

Zone 4: lumbar gluteal muscles and external edge of the sacrum.

Zone 5: region of the buttocks. The caudal femoral muscles (semimembranosus, semitendinosus and biceps femoris).

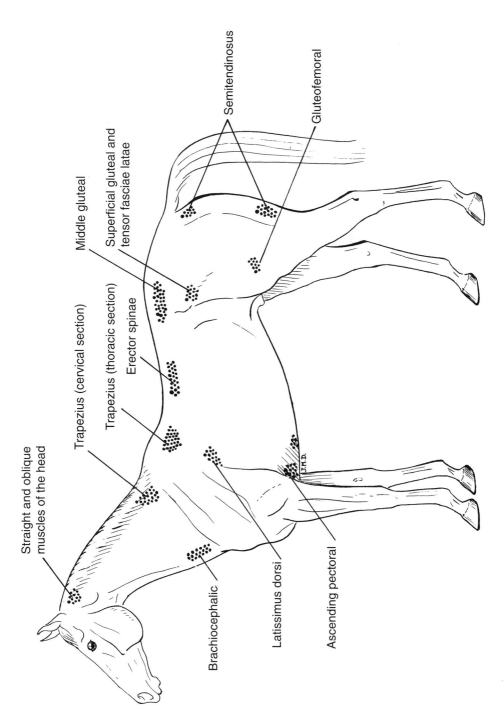

Figure 64 Principal points of tension.

Semitendinosus

Gluteofemoral

Superficial gluteal and tensor fasciae latae

Middle gluteal

Trapezius (cervical section)

Trapezius (thoracic section)

Erector spinae

Straight and oblique muscles of the head

Brachiocephalic

Latissimus dorsi

Ascending pectoral

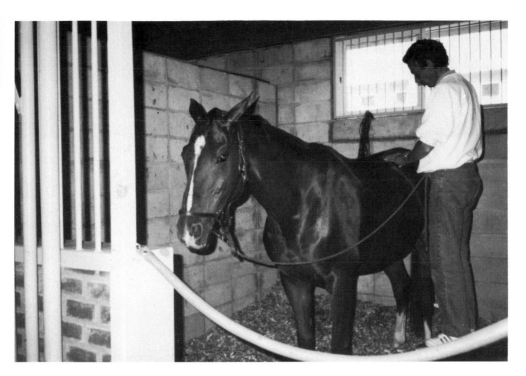

Photo 24 Ilio-lumbar massage.

The interspinous ligaments of all these vertebral zones may require treatment of the following kind: DTM, iontophoresis (with sodium salicylate or potassium iodide), anti-inflammatory drugs.

2.5 PHYSIOTHERAPY OF THE DORSO-LUMBAR AREA

(a) A typical session

1. PRIOR TO MASSAGE

1. Application of thermal mud pack, 30 cm by 25 cm, to the affected area.
2. Low frequency electrotherapy for 15–20 min; 4 electrodes placed on the points of tension (either anode or cathode can be placed on the painful area). Raise the current very gradually, to the point where a light tremor becomes apparent.

2. MASSAGE
See photo 24. Follow principles described above.

3. ULTRASOUND
Some contractions which resist treatment can be relieved using ultrasound; this should be pulsed rather than continuous, set at 35–40 watts, sweep slowly over the tense area, and last 12 min. As a rule, massage should be sufficient to initiate the process of recovery, but there

is no reason why the professional therapist should not achieve success by supplementing this with electrotherapy.

4. REFLEX THERAPY
Acupuncture or any other reflex technique (such as massage) is appropriate when used in conjunction with the therapeutic techniques described above. Treatment sessions should preferably take place in the evening, and once started, should not be interrupted prior to completion. A course of 10 sessions, every two days, is recommended; massage of the acupuncture points, however, should be restricted to 2 or 3 sessions, spaced at intervals of 2 days. These treatments are demanding but are highly effective at promoting recovery.

It is worth reiterating the points raised earlier in this book concerning the care and supervision required by the equine athlete working at the limit of its capabilities. Human athletes have for many years benefited from physiotherapeutic and medical attention; vertebral problems are not left unattended. The horse, however, frequently suffers from similar problems which are poorly comprehended by the rider. Sometimes pain is treated as resistance and the horse penalized – this underlies the improvement seen when some horses change owner.

There is a close interconnection between the limbs and the back; taking care of the former and ignoring the latter results in immediate relapse. The limbs should be checked and the horse's stand corrected to prevent the jarring effect of defects in locomotion ultimately finding their way to the back. Heels which are too low, for example, will strain the musculo-articular framework of the hocks, resulting in resistance in the lumbo-sacral area.

A complete orthopedic examination and diagnosis by a vet specializing in horses is of great importance. Physiotherapy is not a substitute for veterinary attention. It is a complementary therapy, a continuation of medical and surgical treatment.

5. EXERCISES
If the horse is not seriously incapacitated and finding locomotion difficult, but simply experiencing pain and stiffness in its back, it is recommended that the exercise session end with 10 minutes on the lunge, using a chambon with a rubber intermediary. The back should be covered. Care should be taken to start on the less sensitive and more supple side. If necessary, one can restrict the work to this side alone for several days, before changing the incurvation. In cold and damp weather the cover should be left on the horse's back when it returns to its box.

(b) Massage technique
Treatment should take the whole back into account, even if pain has been tracked to a particular, limited area – the paravertebral muscles work together as a chain; one painful link disturbs the whole. However, two regions, dorsal and lumbo-gluteal, can be distinguished. In each of these regions there are special tension points which require treatment to be extended around them.

1. CLASSICAL MASSAGE (photos 25 to 28 and Fig. 65)
The therapist stands beside the horse, on a bale of hay or stool; the lead of the halter can be passed through the trouser belt to keep the patient close by. The session begins with massage extending from the withers to the gluteal region using the flat of the hands. This helps calm the horse and provides the initial 'reading' of its back. The horse should be free to turn its head to watch the massage as it progresses. A little hay can be placed in front of it to persuade it to lower its neck, which will assist the treatment.

By stimulating ventral flexion the sensitivity of the supra- and interspinous ligaments can be assessed. A pronounced swelling around the spinous processes (apophyses) may indicate

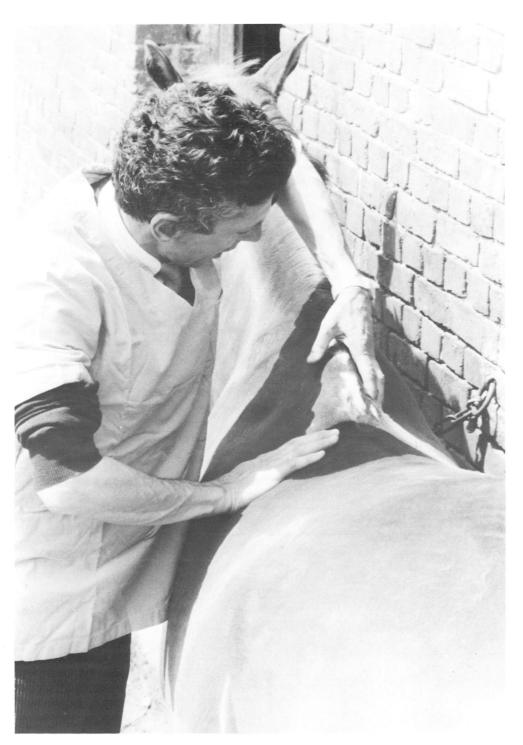

Photo 25 Massage of the trapezius.

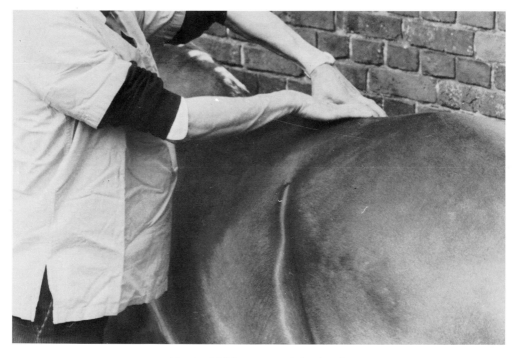

Photo 26 Massage of the back.

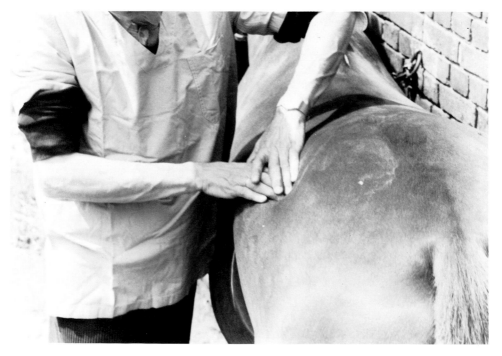

Photo 27 Massage of the back.

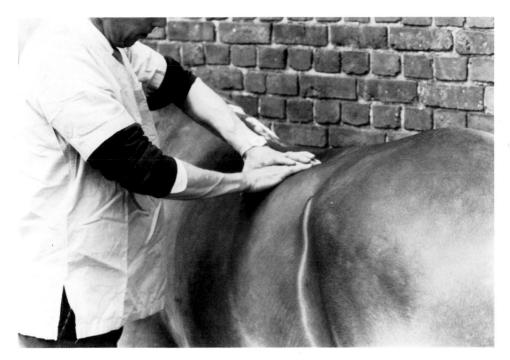

Photo 28 Massage of the back.

OSP; in such cases the peripheral area of the joint is particularly sensitive. Tenderness in the gluteal region can be evidence of lumbago or lumbar sciatica, in which case it will extend as far as the caudal femoral muscles. A series of pinches of the skin to separate the layers is effective in treating both of these conditions, particularly sciatica. If the hairs are standing proud of the skin (horripilation), this can, in some cases, be caused by the impact of strong sunshine on a dermatome, causing sciatica.

Analysis of the various layers of the integument therefore constitutes the first stage of the therapeutic relationship. As the massage becomes more penetrating the therapist stops to 'listen' to the contractions occurring at the deeper levels while treating them with transversal manipulation using the pads of the fingers. One should work slowly, feeling the layers of muscles stretch beneath the fingers, initiating relaxation in the tension points. The therapist moves back and forth between the withers and the croup, attending to each painful area, and then from the attachments of the gluteal muscles at the ilium, along the sacrum towards the tail – very important for the treatment of lumbar problems. When a tense point is identified treatment should continue within the area for 5 minutes. It is preferable to go with the lay of the hair, working longitudinally and transversally, making downward movements beginning at the lateral edge of the spinous processes.

2. REFLEX MASSAGE

When used as a complement to classical massage, reflex treatment of the back according to the schema of lines indicated in Fig. 66 can give good results. This technique is practised during a calm moment, preferably in the evening. Each line is worked 3 times, quite deeply, with the points of the fingers as though one wished to penetrate the skin. Movement along the line is slow, and makes use of the forearm. The strokes used are as follows:

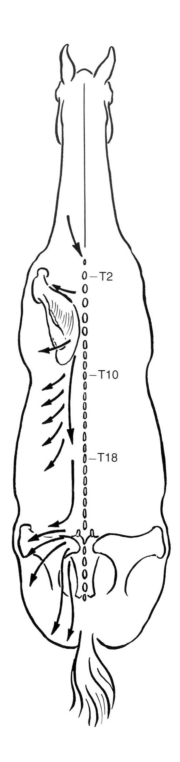

Figure 65 Lines indicating massage strokes on the back and croup.

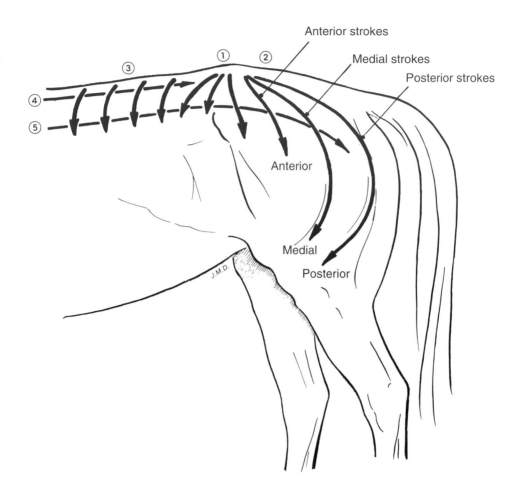

Figure 66 Lines indicating reflex massage strokes on the loins and croup.

1. Fan-shaped strokes in the ilio-lumbar area, between the vertebral column and the insertions of the gluteal muscles, each repeated 3 times.
2. Downward strokes in the gluteal area:
• 3 anterior, towards the angle of the hip or lateral iliac spine;
• 3 median, towards the hip joint;
• 3 posterior, towards the muscular fold commonly called the 'misery line'.
3. Downward oblique strokes in the lumbar area, 10 cm long and spaced 3 to 4 cm apart, from just behind the saddle – 3 times. Work from the ilio-lumbar intersection up to the withers. Repeat the whole treatment 3 times.
4. Longitudinal strokes from front to back – 3 times, 2 cm from the median line of the spinous processes.
5. Antispasmodic strokes from front to back, with the flat of the hand, working simultaneously on both sides, from the middle of the back to the tail, passing over the gluteal muscles.

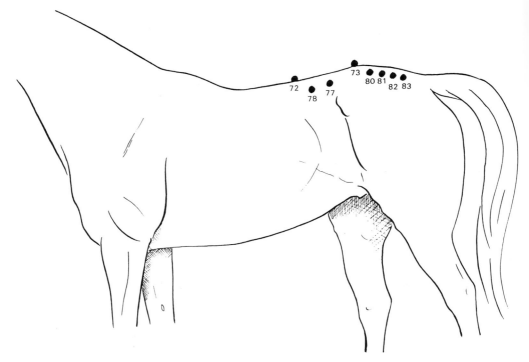

Figure 67 Massage of acupuncture points in the lumbo-gluteal region.

With some horses, massage of the pectoral region (the descending pectoral muscle between the forelimbs) is an important method of inducing relaxation. The horse sometimes becomes so relaxed that it rests its nose on the ground and closes its eyes.

3. MASSAGE OF THE ACUPUNCTURE POINTS (see Fig. 67)

72   location: dorsal median line between the 2nd and 3rd lumbar vertebrae;
        to treat: tendino-muscular pains in the dorso-lumbar region.
73   location: median line between the last lumbar and first sacral vertebrae;
        to treat: all dorso-lumbar pain.
77/78 location: 2 measures (1 measure = 3 cm) away from the median line and 4 and 6
        measures (12 and 18 cm) towards the front;
        to treat: pain, contraction and myositis in the dorso-lumbar region.
80–83 locations:
        80 in a small cavity 3.5 cm away from the median line at the level of the 1st sacral
        vertebra;
        81 in a small cavity between S1 and S2;
        82 in the interspinous space between S2 and S3;
        83 in the interspinous space between S3 and S4;
        to treat: pain in the lumbo-sacral area and weakness in the kidney area.

Conclude with a penetrating linear massage between 80 and 83; make several passes with the points of the fingers simultaneously on each side.

2.6 VERTEBRAL RE-EDUCATION

Re-education should follow massage and electrotherapy. Its aim, in the initial stage, is to reinforce the abdominal musculature and strengthen flexion of the vertebral bridge. Attention is then given to restoring the tonus of the extensor muscles in harmony with dorsal and ventral tensions.

(a) Programme

1. Rein-back, in hand, at walking pace up an incline 10 to 15 metres long, without raising the neck.
2. Volte, in hand, at walking pace, 5–10 voltes on each rein.
3. Work on the lunge with incurvation and lowering of the neck, the circle 10 metres in diameter and 4 poles on the ground.
4. Canter on the lunge, initially with a slow, relaxed, unhurried gait, the neck low; then lift both the chest and neck, which balances and shortens the stride.
5. Conclude the session by mounting the horse and perform the following exercises:
- work on two tracks at the three gaits;
- a series of successive changes in pace – walk, canter, walk – without losing equilbrium while changing from one to the other. This provides support for the back;
- rein-back;
- false or counter canter, which also helps to strengthen the back;
- figure eight, half at a false canter; develop engagement while executing the canter on the correct lead.

At all times, the rider should check his or her position on the horse's vertebral bridge. If rein-back is performed using exaggerated movements of the upper body, it increases the weight on the thoraco-lumbar region and affects the horse's equilibrium. If, however, the rider can maintain an upright position in the saddle, not only will the equilibrium be unaffected but an excess of weight on the thoraco-lumbar hinge joint will also be avoided.

The walk and the canter are the two gaits which are most useful for the development of vertebral mobility and suppleness. By directing the horse in hand around oneself at a slow and arrhythmic walk, one can stimulate movement of the vertebral joints. This should be done prior to mounting a horse suffering from back problems. This exercise provides the rider with the opportunity to examine the flexions and rotations of the back while it is unencumbered. It opens the intervertebral spaces; it stretches the ligaments around the joints and also the deeper, cybernetic muscles around the vertebral column. Having been 'woken up' in this way, the back is in a better condition to adapt to the displacements caused by the weight of the rider. Two to three minutes on each rein is sufficient preparation for a horse just out of its box, with a cold and stiff back. Stretching of the muscles and ligaments will avoid the reflex contractions caused by a cold back which can persist throughout the whole session. A great many potentially chronic thoraco-lumbar problems originate at this stage.

(b) Preparatory work on the lunge
This work, which proceeds in two stages, helps strengthen and consolidate the vertebral-abdominal connection.

1. STRETCHING AND RELAXATION OF THE DORSAL MUSCULO-ARTICULAR CHAIN

1. Using the side reins the neck should be pointed downwards so that the nose is level with the knees.
2. Work at the trot for 5 min on each rein.
3. Place 3 bars on the ground, 1 to 2 metres apart, to develop the cadence of the trot and work the thoraco-lumbar hinge joint.
4. Vigorously maintain cadence, which is a very important contributor to the freedom and suppleness of movement. Cadence reflects the horse's state of relaxation, easing the movement of joints and expanding the amplitude of movement of the spine.

During this essential first stage, the slow tempo and cadence of the trot, and the position of the neck, help provide the following:

1. Release of paravertebral tensions.
2. Amplification of vertebral movement.
3. Development of the external layer of the lumbo-caudal muscles involved in propulsion, particularly the mid-gluteal.
4. Activation of the abdominal region which assists lumbar relaxation.

2. RESTORING THE TONICITY AROUND THE POINT OF EQUILIBRIUM

1. Using the side reins, flex the neck and raise it so that it is in its usual position.
2. Work at the trot for 5 min on each rein.
3. Maintain a regular cadence.
4. Do not use cavalettis.
5. Inititiate several strike-offs at the canter from walking pace.
6. Conclude with 15 voltes at a canter, on each rein.

This session will help restore muscular equilibrium between the 'top' and 'bottom' lines (as described in Chapter 2, pages 57, 61). The canter helps tone the abdominal muscles and the hinge joint supporting the middle gluteal muscle which is the anchorage point holding the dorsal chain in position. Thirty min after this preparatory work, the horse can be worked while mounted.

(c) Physiotherapeutic analysis of work with the neck lowered
The following biomechanic and physiotherapeutic analysis of working with the neck lowered concentrates on its impact on three major regions of the body: forehand, trunk and hindquarters (see photo 29).

1. FOREHAND
Whatever the gait, be it walk, trot or canter, lowering of the neck introduces several modifications to the usual biomechanical functioning of this area.

The most visible consequence is the increased loading that it bears, which is paralleled by the simultaneous lightening of the load on the hindquarters, due to the centre of gravity being shifted forwards by leverage exerted by the cervico-cephalic region. The consequent overloading increases the work of the muscular girdles and results in the raising of the chest area between the two forelimbs. The development of the pectoral and serratus muscles

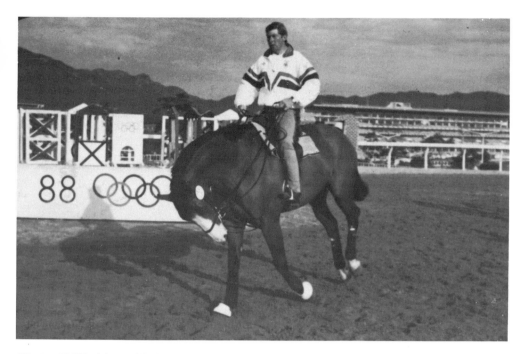

Photo 29 Working with the neck lowered strengthens the abdominal muscles and relaxes the 'top' line.

contributes to improved support and makes the forequarters lighter when the neck is returned to its normal position.

While this exercise undeniably contributes towards performance, it must not be practised too often, nor be prolonged, as the overloading increases pressures on the joints and tendons in the forelimbs. It is therefore counter-indicated for horses with a past record of tendinitis or joint disease.

Lowering the neck also works on the dorsal cervical muscles as they respond to the increase in leverage. The external part of the muscles contract isometrically. This action has dual benefits in that it both helps contain the eventual muscular spasms and increases the effectiveness of contraction. The muscles most directly involved are those which mobilize the cervico-thoracic junction, i.e. those situated at the base of the neck and in the cranial thoracic region. The development of these muscles and the cervico-cephalic levator muscles, which extend the neck and raise the forehand after the forelimbs touch the ground, make the exercise of obvious interest to those competing in dressage and jumping.

Finally, lowering the neck also opens the intervertebral foramina (the gaps between neighbouring vertebra which allow the passage of spinal nerves where they connect to the spinal cord). This helps relieve pain due to constrictions or irritations which can translate itself into stiffness in the back or lameness in the forelimbs.

2. TRUNK

As a rule, lowering the neck causes flexion of the thoracic spine, simultaneously stretching and elongating the area above the vertebral axis and causing an increase in work in the abdominal muscles below it. However, the constraints and effects vary if the the hindquarters are either simultaneously engaged or not.

2.1 Without engagement

Effects on the vertebrae and vertebral ligaments
Lowering brings about the separation of the spinous processes along the length of the thoracic spine; as this is an analgesic posture for horses suffering from OSP it therefore constitutes an effective physiotherapeutic treatment regime for this condition. The strong traction exerted by the nuchal ligament on the very high spinous processes at the withers causes a parallel flexion along the thoracic spine, particularly between T6 and T10. This vertebral curve, as our research since 1984 has shown, occurs in the area of the saddle, directly below the rider. It helps bring about an elevation of the back and facilitates carrying the weight of the rider, which is of particular benefit to young horses which have not developed the musculature to bear this load, or to horses with OSP, for which every extension brings pain.

Effects on the muscles of the back
Lowering the neck influences the muscles and ligaments situated above the vertebral axis as far as the thoraco-lumbar junction. The vertebral curve also induces stretching of the powerful erector spinae group and of the juxtavertebral muscles which lengthen as a result. As this improves the effectiveness of muscular contraction, it is of obvious interest to trainers. The stretching has the additional benefit of containing secondary reflex contractions which are associated with numerous back problems such as OSP and arthrosis of the dorsal synovial joints.

2.2 With engagement
Thoracic flexion caused by lowering is accompanied by the supraspinous ligament being placed under tension. The horse must counter the tension if it is to engage the hind limbs. This has competitive benefits and drawbacks.

Benefits
These are as described above. However, constraint on flexion at both extremities of the spinal column presents additional benefits. Engagement increases the flexion of the thoraco-lumbar vertebral bridge so effectively that the biomechanical consequences are more pronounced. In the thoracic region, the separation of the spinous processes, the vertebral curve beneath the rider and the stretching of the erector spinae and juxtavertebral muscles are further intensified. As the tensioning of the supraspinous ligament reduces the possibilities for flexion of the lumbar spine, the following positive modifications occur:

1. *Muscular.* For the hindlimbs to be engaged, the abdominal muscles must work harder to counter the effect of the non-stretching of the ligament in the lumbar region. This helps to promote their development. The muscles can be divided into two groups: (i) the straight and oblique muscles of the abdominal wall and (ii) the psoas and iliac muscles on the ventral side of the vertebral column.
2. *Vertebral.* During flexion and extension there is forward stretching of the supraspinous ligament produced by the traction of the nuchal ligament; there is also backward stretching produced by the abdominal muscles. This helps make the spine more supple.
3. Limitations placed on flexion of the lumbar spine are compensated by lateral flexion and rotation. As we have already seen in Chapter 2, these movements chiefly involve the lower thoracic spine; they are of little importance in the lumbar and lumbo-sacral areas. The muscles involved in acting on the latter are essentially the oblique internal and external muscles in the abdomen and the juxtavertebral muscles. The combination of movements

and the muscular interventions associated with them when the horse is worked with the neck lowered contribute to the increased mobility of the column in all directions.

Drawbacks
Despite all these advantages, practice of this exercise must be limited, due to biomechanical resistance of various parts of the spine. Excess of tension can cause:

1. Lesions on the supraspinous ligament and its attachments, resulting in periostitis and desmitis.
2. Lesions on the vertebral bodies and intervertebral discs brought about by a parallel increase in compression.

3. EFFECTS ON THE HINDQUARTERS
Lowering the neck not only affects the equilibrium of the horse, completely upsetting the vertebral mechanism, it also appears to have repercussions on the functioning of the hindquarters, and (of consequence to competitive performance) the lumbo-sacral and coxo-femoral joints.

3.1 Lumbo-sacral joint
Recent research which we have carried out at the Veterinary School of Lyon (Laboratory of Research on the Horse in Competition) indicates that lowering the neck is accompanied by a reduction in lumbar mobility, but that increased involvement in flexion by the lumbo-sacral joint when the hindquarters are engaged helps to offset this. (The absence, in this area of the spine, of the supraspinous ligament and the relative weakness of the interspinous ligament are also helpful.) The increase in lumbo-sacral flexion has the following benefits for equitation:

1. The joint becomes more supple as a result of the continued muscular tension.
2. Assisted by a downward tilting of the pelvis, traction is exerted on the powerful erector spinae muscles (rearwards) and on the mid-gluteal muscles (forwards). These large muscular groups, which provide the main motive force in impulsion, are thus stretched to the maximum while they work.
3. The work rate of the muscles involved in lumbar and lumbo-sacral flexion is increased, thus helping to develop them. These muscles, which we have mentioned several times already, are the rectus and obliquus in the abdominal wall, and the iliopsoas in the sub-lumbar region. The latter terminates on the femur and has a direct impact on the mobility of the hip joint.

3.2 Joints of the hip and hindlimb
The tension exerted by the iliopsoas when it counters the reduction in lumbar mobility is applied to the upper extremity of the femur. As a consequence, as each hindlimb is engaged, hip flexion is increased. When engagement is combined with lumbo-sacral flexion, it stretches the gluteal muscles, and when synchronized with the extension of the stifle joint, the femoral caudal muscles (biceps femoris, semitendinosus and semimembranosus). The movements of the joints thereby become involved in the elongation of all the muscles involved in impulsion, which enhances strength and power in jumping.

These multiple benefits make working with the neck lowered one of the main exercises for both physical preparation and re-education.

(d) Biomechanical effects of exercises with the neck lowered

1. STRETCHING OF THE MUSCLES AND LIGAMENTS IN THE DORSAL CHAIN

1. Tensioning of the supra- and interspinous ligaments.
2. Lengthening of the chain.

2. MOBILIZATION OF THE VERTEBRAL JOINTS
This is brought about by:

1. Working the superficial and deep paravertebral muscles in a way that enhances the opening up of the joints.
2. Rhythmic trotting accompanied by changes in pace, which works on the joints and muscles.

The following benefits are particularly liberating, prophylactic and therapeutic for the back:

1. Freeing up of the dorso-lumbar area.
2. Stretching of the muscles and ligaments.
3. Alternating tensions in the paravertebral muscles.
4. Gentle axial rotation of the vertebrae (when trotting diagonally).

3. REINFORCEMENT OF THE 'BOTTOM' LINE
Strengthening (shorterning of the fibres of) the abdominal and iliopsoas muscles.

4. SYNERGY OF THE GLUTEAL AND CAUDAL FEMORAL MUSCLES

1. The effect on the middle gluteal muscle, with its lumbar anchorage point, is particularly interesting.
2. The caudal femoral muscles are stretched while working, which enhances the quality of the muscle fibres.

3. ADDITIONAL PARVERTEBRAL PATHOLOGIES IN THE TRUNK

3.1 SACRO-ILIAC JOINT

When subjected to trauma or arthrosis, pain can radiate from the joint into the surrounding gluteal and caudal femoral muscles, causing spasms and lameness.

(a) Treatment

1. Deep massage of the muscles along the sacrum, and in the sacro-iliac space (see photo 30).
2. Excitomotor (faradic) electrotherapy, lasting 30 min, applied to the insertions of the gluteal and sacro-iliac muscles.
3. Ultrasound applied in and around the sacro-iliac space, and to the insertions of the sacro-iliac muscles;

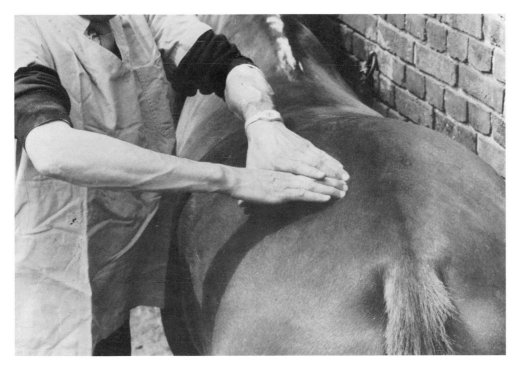

Photo 30 Massage of the sacro-iliac area.

4. Conclude with cutaneous stimulation, causing 5 or 6 ventral flexions. After this, the horse is led on a volte of 2 to 3 metres; work the lumbo-sacral joint and attempt maximum engagement of the muscles on the inside of the hindlimb, which causes contralateral stretching of the external muscular chain.

3.2 FALSE LAMENESS (IRREGULARITIES IN THE GAIT)

False lameness is defined as a breakdown in muscular synergy in the dorso-lumbar and pelvic areas. It manifests itself as an intermittent irregularity in the gait, which disappears during cadence and impulsion.

(a) Origins

1. Lack of strength in the upper muscular chain.
2. Muscular disengagement, or breakdown in continuity due to musculo-vertebral problems.
3. Sequelae of myositis.
4. Developing OSP, with signs of pain in the intervertebral areas.
5. Cybernetic conflict due to cramps in the multifidus muscles.

(b) Treatment

1. Physiotherapeutic treatment of lumbar and dorso-lumbar problems.
2. Re-education:
- Regular, reassuring hand contact.
- Slowing down of cadence.
- More positive impulsion.
- Orienting the work towards collection without abrupt changes and with increased confidence.
- Feeling when the rhythm is pain-free and working with it.
- Inhibiting expansive movement.
- Temporary reduction of work on two tracks while the horse is still unable to provide sufficient support for its back.

3.3 DORSO-LUMBAR MYOSITIS

This inflammation arises as a result of problems in muscle tissue metabolism.

(a) Aetiology
Several factors appear to be involved in the genesis of this condition:

1. Nutrition.
2. Irregular rhythm of work – sessions which are too intense followed by rest periods which are too long.
3. Transportation which is either prolonged, unusual or stress-producing.
4. Climatic conditions – excess of heat or cold.

(b) Symptoms
When these are intense their impact on the psoas muscles is so brutal that the whole lumbar-pelvic area is reduced almost immediately to impotence. The 'loins' of the horse are locked, preventing any movement of the lumbar spine. In some cases it can affect other muscular groups, e.g. caudal femoral muscles and triceps brachii. Certain sequelae of sciatica present a comparable picture: the gluteal and caudal femoral muscles become 'boxed-in' and painful, with a sub-cutaneous inflammatory infiltrate. These are the reactions of the myotome to the radiculalgia (pain in the spinal nerves) caused by the sciatica. The dermatome, which is connected to the myotome, reacts to this inflammation.

(c) Physiotherapeutic treatment
The first prescription is immediate and total rest for the patient, lasting 3 days. The initial treatment begins on the 4th day and is repeated every subsequent day for 2 weeks.

1. APPLICATION OF THERMAL MUD
The mud is warmed to 50°C; this temperature is maintained by returning the pack to a bowl filled with hot water. Each application, about 30 cm wide, is placed on the back of the horse at the lumbo-gluteal junction above T10. It is applied for 30–45 min.

2. ELECTROTHERAPY

Low frequency excitomotor (faradic) currents are used. The frequency is set at 30 to 80Hz and applied with low intensity until a tremor of the muscular layer starts to become apparent. Some compact machines have 4 electrodes, allowing the therapist to position 2 in the dorso-lumbar region between T15 and T18 and a further 2 in the lumbar-gluteal region in the angle formed by the ilium and lumbar spine.

3. MASSAGE

This is performed immediately after electrotherapy. The initial stage is classical massage of the dorso-lumbar muscles, working largely on the paravertebral layer from the withers as far as the buttocks. This is followed by massage of the gluteal muscles (sacro-iliac triangle). The session concludes with massage of the caudal femoral muscles using the petrissage technique and shaking of the muscular bodies. The session should last for 20–30 min.

4. RE-EDUCATION

This follows immediately after the massage, but should not be undertaken unless one is certain that there is no attendant discomfort. The back of the horse should be covered during the first sessions. Begin by leading the horse at the walk for a few minutes.

The following programme is proposed as a guide, and can be altered according to the horse's rate of clinical recovery:

- *Day 1:* 5 min walk;
- *Days 2–4:* add 5 min to the walk each day;
- *Day 5:* work on the lunge twice a day – 5 min walk, 5 min trot;
- *Days 6–14:* increase walk and trot by 2–3 min each day;

- *Starting at Day 15*

Mounted work should not begin before Day 15 and should always be preceded by warming up on the lunge – 5 min walk, 5 min trot. Mounted work at the trot should be suspended for one week in order to prevent the back being overloaded and to allow the joints to function unencumbered. Cantering sessions should be interrupted by brief rest periods lasting 1–2 min. Work on two tracks should be left until the previous exercises reveal definite signs of improvement. After mounted work the session should always conclude with 15 min on the lunge, at a walk, with the neck free. Relapses should always be watched for, so the following conditions are obligatory:

1. Regularity during work sessions.
2. No rest days.
3. Feeding according to requirements to avoid excesses of energy.
4. Blanket on the back when weather is cold or damp during the first 15 min of warming up exercises and final 15 min of work on the lunge.

4. THE SHOULDER

4.1 INTRODUCTION

The shoulders carry 60% of the weight of the Horse.

Each shoulder-joint is closely fastened to the rib-cage by the serratus and pectoral muscles. Two biomechanical forces are transmitted to it: the response to gravity and the momentum imparted by the thrusting of the hindquarters. Due to its mobility and oblique positioning the joint provides the amplitude of movement which enables the forelimb to negotiate the ground in front of it. It also works together with the tendons in the digits and the suspensory ligament in the pastern to provide a shock absorption system which is particularly valuable for competitive obstacle jumping. During extension the pectoral muscles impart to the forelimb a light adductive tightening in relation to the median axis.

Lameness in the shoulder has a tendency to be a 'catch-all' for a variety of problems. Identification of the true causes – which include deep lacerations, tendinitis of the extensors of the arm and lesions in the trapezius – requires a meticulous and searching examination; in this context it is important to emphasize again the *effectiveness* of palpation. Various lesions can be located, none of which are easy to treat on their own because they are all inter-connected. With careful treatment, the shoulder will recover in spite of this, but slowly; it does not present a clear picture of recovery on the path to resumption of normal locomotion. It is only after 3 or 4 weeks of work on the flat, without any sign of lameness, that resumption of jumping should be contemplated.

However, this prudent, gradualist approach is frequently not adopted; consequently, painful lapses are frequent and this ailment has a poor reputation. It is the shoulder's role in shock absorption which makes it so vulnerable, and why the watchwords for re-education are 'go gently, slow down, redevelop the muscles'.

4.2 KEY POINTS IN THE SHOULDER

These are indicated in Fig. 68.

(a) Supraspinatus

1. Extensor of the arm, 'locking' the shoulder when the forelimb lands.
2. Discomfort is exhibited when the forelimb connects with the ground and when the arm is extended.
3. Lesions occur in two areas: the middle quarter of the muscle and the tendon where it connects with the shoulder joint.

(b) Infraspinatus

1. Flexor and abductor of the arm, also involved in 'locking' the shoulder.
2. Discomfort is exhibited when the area is touched, as well as during flexion and abduction.
3. Sites of lesions as for supraspinatus (the tendon less frequently).

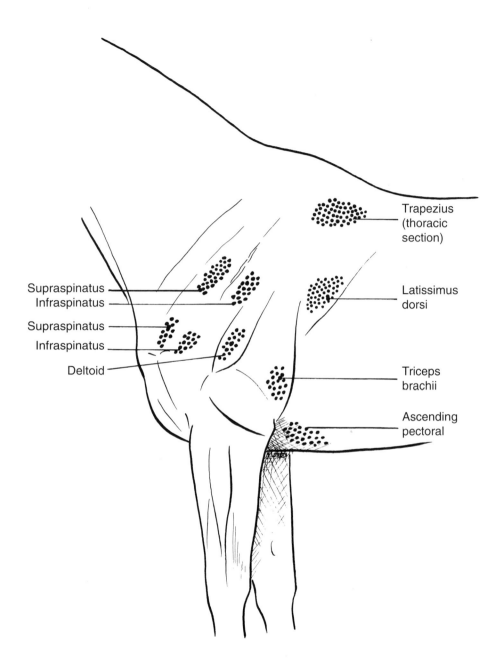

Supraspinatus

Infraspinatus

Supraspinatus

Infraspinatus

Deltoid

Trapezius
(thoracic
section)

Latissimus
dorsi

Triceps
brachii

Ascending
pectoral

Figure 68 Key points in the shoulder.

(c) Deltoid

1. Flexor and abductor of the arm, offers lateral consolidation and support to the shoulder.
2. Pathology in this area is frequently due to the horse struggling against confinement, e.g. in the box or trailer.
3. Rupture is apparent from a drop in the position of the elbow (which distinguishes this condition from radial paralysis).

(d) Triceps brachii

1. This is polyarticular (crosses more than one joint), fulfilling a double role as flexor of the shoulder and extensor of the elbow. It cushions the shoulder during landing and 'locks' the elbow. It is also involved in impulsion.
2. If the shoulder is lame, check the areas where the muscle is connected to the joints.

(e) Biceps brachii

1. This is also polyarticular, involved in extension of the shoulder and flexion of the forearm. It is active in 'locking' during impulsion, working synergistically with the caudal muscles of the arm to support the shoulder and elbow.
2. Lesions can be found when the muscle contracts and in inflamed areas in the junction between muscle and tendon.

(f) Serratus and pectoral muscles

1. Their involvement in the support of the scapular girdle in the trunk means that they come under considerable pressure when the forelimbs land, and suffer injury as a result. The larger serratus works together with the brachiocephalic during extension of the arm in order to tilt the shoulder blade.
2. Avoid tight and non-elastic girths which lead to paralysis in the pectoral muscles, as well as problems with circulation (sudden rushes of blood). Palpation of the pectorals will frequently identify hypersensitivity in the ascending pectoral.

(g) Trapezius

1. Together with the rhomboid this muscle forms the dorsal part of the muscular belt around the scapula.
2. It can be directly affected by spasms, or undergo reflex contractions via resonance.

Palpation of the shoulder muscles frequently reveals emotional conflict. As the muscular bodies are very firm and not malleable, one should watch for painful reactions when locating tense areas. Palpating the same muscles on the other side, and comparing the response, enables one to establish the differences in sensitivity and states of tension.

4.3 CARE AND TREATMENT OF THE SHOULDER

For lesions of a strictly muscular nature, such as lacerations or strong contractions, refer to the previous chapter. Alternatively, one can put into effect the following schedule of treatments for shoulder-specific complaints.

(a) General schedule

1. *Rest.* During the initial days, complete rest.
2. *Cooling* of the insertions of the tendons if tendinitis is diagnosed; shower the area with a fine jet of water to avoid wetting other parts of the body.
3. *Massage* of the muscular body near to the affected tendon.
4. *Electrotherapy.* Apply medium frequency current for 15 min to the affected muscle and joint. Interferential therapy can also be used for the trapezius muscles; this involves placing an electrode on either side of the withers and large plates further down towards the scapula.
5. *Ultrasound.* Without provoking a sensitive reaction, apply for 12 min to the affected muscle and tendon; sweep over the area where the tendon terminates, using pulses.

(b) Re-education

This should follow the treatments listed above.

1. While the horse is still in its box, stretch the shoulder in order to mobilize it. Place the forelimb in front of the horse and in a series of gentle movements flex it and move it sideways for 5 min.
2. Lead the horse out of the box and exercise it on the lunge with side-reins; the neck should be lifted so as not to overload the forehand.
3. Exercise on the volte on the side of the lesion, at walking pace, for several days before breaking into a trot. The formation of scar tissue requires that the area not be subjected to shocks. The ground should be regular and flat, and above all, not hard.
4. At the start of mounted work, begin with a light rider who can maintain balance and not exercise the forehand *at all*.
5. There should be no cantering, and no work with the opposing incurvation before 8 to 15 days.
6. When returning from work there is a choice of treatments depending on whether the problem is tendinitis or laceration. For the former, use of an ice-pack; for the latter, drainage massage for 10 min.

(c) Massage

This is required in the following circumstances:

1. Trauma, resulting from the horse being wedged in its box or thrown against the side of the trailer; also due to poor landing following a jump.
2. Overwork or muscular fatigue derived from participation in 3-day events or from overextension during dressage.

While the horse is in a resting position, muscle tensioning and acupuncture massage can be used (see photos 31 and 32) in addition to classical techniques.

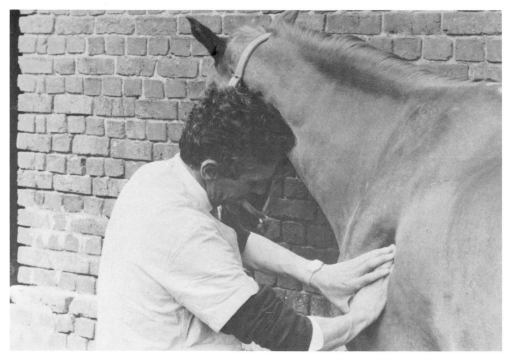

Photo 31 Massage of the shoulder.

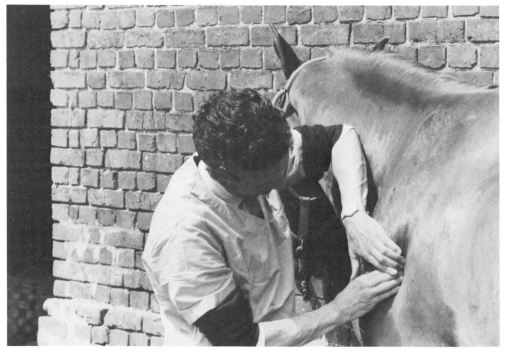

Photo 32 Massage of the shoulder.

1. MUSCLE TENSIONING MASSAGE

The physiological justification for this technique is as follows:

1. When the neuromuscular spindles are placed under tension, the defensive mechanisms of the muscle generate a spasticity which is more rapidly relieved when the area is simultaneously stretched and massaged.
2. The Golgi mechanoreceptors located at the junction between muscle and tendon are also placed under tension by the stretching.
3. The fascias and fibrous tissue adapt to the tension after about 6 seconds of stretching. This has the effect of relieving spasms. Relief is due to the fact that the fibrous partitions in and around the muscles adapt more slowly to the stretching than the muscle bodies themselves.

See Figs. 69, 70 and 71 and photo 33 for massage technique while stretching. This technique should only be practised once the muscles have had a chance to warm up. It should *never* be practised at the beginning of treatment. It is specifically recommended for use after work, or as part of re-education; it can also be carried out on the evening before important jumping competitions and 3-day events. The practitioner instructs an assistant who positions and stretches the limb, and also periodically relaxes it partially during the massage. During these relaxation phases, the massage is more penetrating, although care is taken not to cause pain.

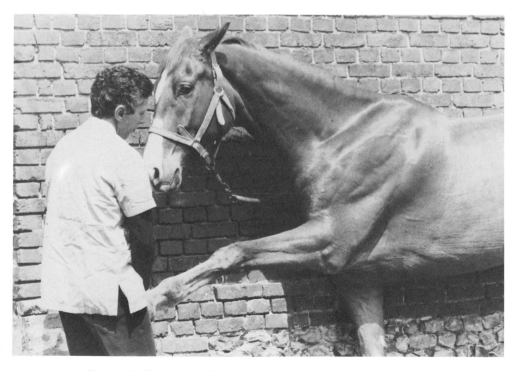

Photo 33 Stretching the propulsor muscles in the shoulder.

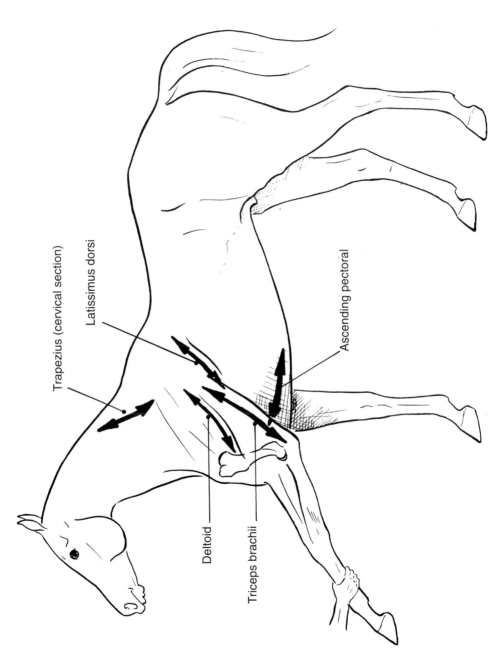

Trapezius (cervical section)

Latissimus dorsi

Ascending pectoral

Deltoid

Triceps brachii

Figure 69 Protraction of the forelimb, showing lengthened muscles and massage areas.

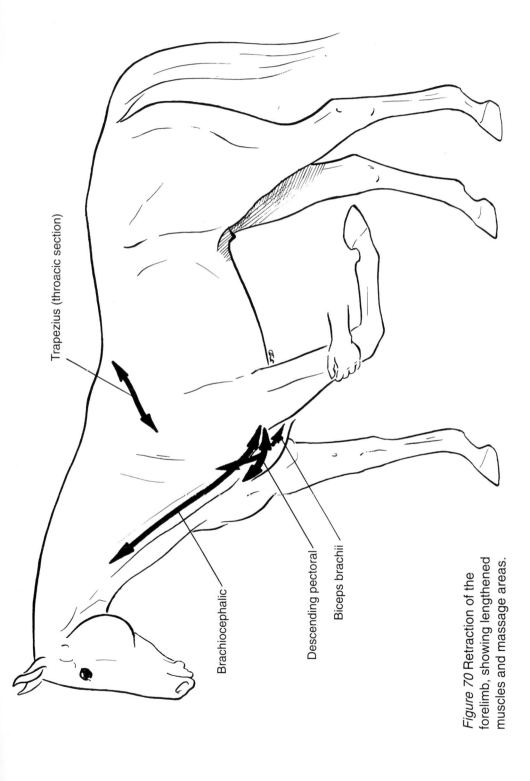

Trapezius (throacic section)

Brachiocephalic

Descending pectoral

Biceps brachii

Figure 70 Retraction of the forelimb, showing lengthened muscles and massage areas.

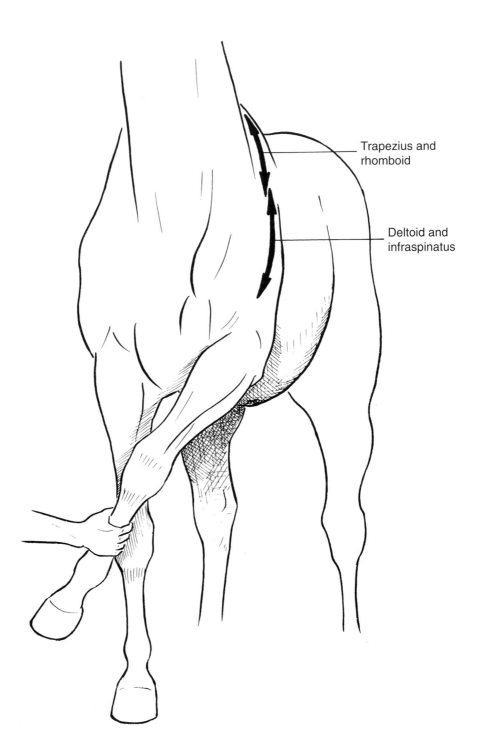

Trapezius and
rhomboid

Deltoid and
infraspinatus

Figure 71 Adduction of the forelimb, showing lengthening of lateral shoulder
        muscles.

2. MASSAGE OF THE ACUPUNCTURE POINTS IN THE SHOULDER
These are illustrated in Fig. 72.

37 location: small cavity in the dorso-cranial angle of the scapula, at the junction with the cartilage;
   to treat: arthritis of the shoulder, paralysis of the scapular nerves, rheumatism in the forelimbs.
38 location: small cavity in the dorso-caudal angle of the scapula, at the junction with the cartilage;
   to treat: same as 37.

2.1 Massaging both points simultaneously

40 location: cranial edge of the scapula, 4 measures below 37 (mid-neck);
   to treat: rheumatism in the shoulder and forelimb, respiratory problems.
39 location: anterior edge of the scapula, 2 measures below 37;
   to treat: arthroses in the shoulder and elbow, paralysis of the scapular nerve, myositis of the sterno- and brachiocephalic.
41 location: small cavity, midway along the caudal edge of the scapula, 4 measures below 38;
   to treat: same as 39.
42 location: angle of the shoulder, small cavity in the upper-anterior edge of the greater tubercle in the humerus;
   to treat: same as 39.
43 location: angle of the shoulder, small cavity in the inferior edge of the greater tubercle;
   to treat: myositis in the brachiocephalic, pain in the shoulder joints.
44 location: depression in the posterior edge of the greater tubercle;
   to treat: same as 43.
45 location: small cavity on the posterior edge of the humerus between the two heads of the deltoid muscle;
   to treat: myositis in this area.
46 location: 3 measures behind 45;
   to treat: contraction of the shoulder muscles and rheumatism in the shoulder.

3. OBSTACLE JUMPING AND THE SHOULDER OF THE HORSE
Landing after jumping an obstacle requires an intense effort by the scapular muscles to 'lock' the scapular girdle and arm. In a high level competition a horse may be required to negotiate all types of terrain or undergo a testing long-distance race with a variety of obstacles; the day after, one can observe painful contractions in the triceps, deltoid, supra- and infraspinatus muscles. Palpation of these muscles can reveal surprisingly high sensitivity, with some horses shrinking away from even the slightest touch. The evening before the trials of a long distance event, such as steeplechase or cross-country, 10 min periscapular massage of both shoulders is recommended. This can be practised again in the morning, some hours before the closing trials begin. Following the evening session there is clear relaxation of the muscles, while the morning session enhances the possibility of almost complete recuperation before the trials. One should in addition remember that the gain in suppleness will help avoid overloading the cushioning provided by the ligaments and tendons.

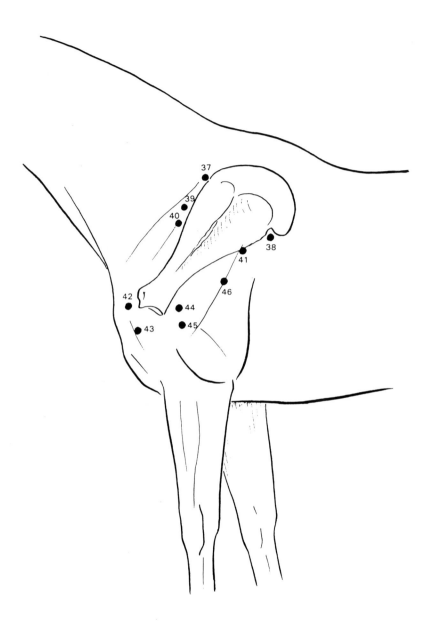

Figure 72 Acupuncture points in the shoulder.

3.1 Additional hints on technique

1. Massage each muscular body within the group affected by the jolting movements of the shoulder.
2. Follow this with stretching of the forelimbs, first raising them and then pulling them backwards.
3. Conclude with another massage.

5. PELVIS AND THIGH

5.1 GENERAL SYMPTOMS

(a) Functional signs
The musculature of this area is involved in propulsion, and painful reactions are frequently seen during the phases of engagement and support, indicating lumbar sciatica. A limb's range of movement is limited as lengthening the caudal muscles becomes painful. At the moment when the limb is poised at the inception of propulsion the muscles are subject to biomechanical constraints which place a brake on the stride and priming of the thrust as it reaches forward.

(b) Diagnosis by palpation
The first area to be examined is around the upper insertions of the middle gluteal muscle. This triangular-shaped tension zone, which appears following contractions of the common lumbar mass, extends laterally to the external protuberance of the ilium and follows the outer edge of the sacrum within the gluteofemoral muscle fibres. It is treated by a series of massages which isolate the various contractions which occur in cases of lumbago and, in particular, sciatica. The latter has a variety of musculo-cutaneous symptoms, which include:

1. Hypersensitivity of the skin covering the posterior external side of the thigh.
2. The skin develops a 'cardboard' quality, becoming extremely sensitive to touch; the horse shrinks away from attempts to mobilize the area beneath the fingers.

In addition to exploring this area, one often finds tension in the caudal femoral semi-membranosus and semitendinosus.

The muscles are also sources of information on vertebral problems and sciatic irritation of the pathological area. Palpating, observing musculo-cutaneous trophism and testing for irritation are all part of a delicate forensic system.

5.2 GENERAL TREATMENT METHODS

(a) Massotherapy
Massotherapy is the name given to the treatment of diseases and disorders by massage.

(b) Re-education
Re-education after massotherapy must be practised according to the following principles:

1. Work is performed on the pain-free side, which is better able to support it, for 75% of the time.

2. A lowered neck is essential; a chambon should be used; slow trot on the lunge, without engagement, so that impulsion is just maintained. The gait should not be 'pushed' beyond this, for 10 to 15 days.
3. From the 10th day, ascents can be made at walking pace, on soft ground.
4. From the 15th day, cavalettis, with the bars placed on the ground to avoid lifting the limbs too much, provide a useful exercise for re-educating the muscles as they adjust to variations in lengthening.
5. Allowing the horse uninhibited movement during the treatment period is forbidden, for this can lead to poorly coordinated and executed movements that can be damaging and traumatizing for the whole musculo-articular system.

5.3 POINTS OF TENSION IN THE REGION

(a) Middle gluteal (see Fig. 73)
Pain in this area is indicative of both lumbar and femoral pathology. Excitomotor electrotherapy and massage are used to treat it. From the point of view of technique, use of the elbow is effective provided that it follows massage with the flat of the hand. The acupuncture points in this area can also be treated, with excellent results.

(b) Semitendinosus
As the muscle fibres lengthen during engagement, tension due to pathology in this area rapidly interferes with locomotion. Pain is also apparent during propulsion, as the muscle body affected by spasms contracts. As indicated in Fig. 73 there are two key tension points, in the upper caudal part of the muscle and in the lower third. The muscular body can be the source of isolated myositis, or it can be implicated in lumbar sciatalgia. During the inflammatory phase, the muscle can take on a cordiform (heart-shaped) appearance, which is accompanied by contractions and loss of suppleness and elasticity.

1. RE-EDUCATION

1. Deep, mobilizing massage using circular movements, 15 min.
2. Ascent, at a walk.
3. Stretching of the dorso-lumbar muscular chain by working with the neck lowered, without engagement.
4. No canter until clinical symptoms have gone and contractions ceased. Work at this gait should initially concentrate on the forelimbs, with the rein on the side opposite the lesion.
5. Use of cavalettis included at the trot during the remuscularization phase.

(c) Semimembranosus (see photo 34)
The tension points are located either in the upper insertion of the muscle or at the junction between the middle and lower thirds. Palpation of the painful points sometimes causes the croup and tail to move away from the therapist. Treatment is the same as for semitendinosus.

(d) Gluteobiceps
This is formed from the fusion of the the cranial part of the biceps and the gluteofemoral muscles. The two heads are equally involved in propulsion and form part of the myofascial

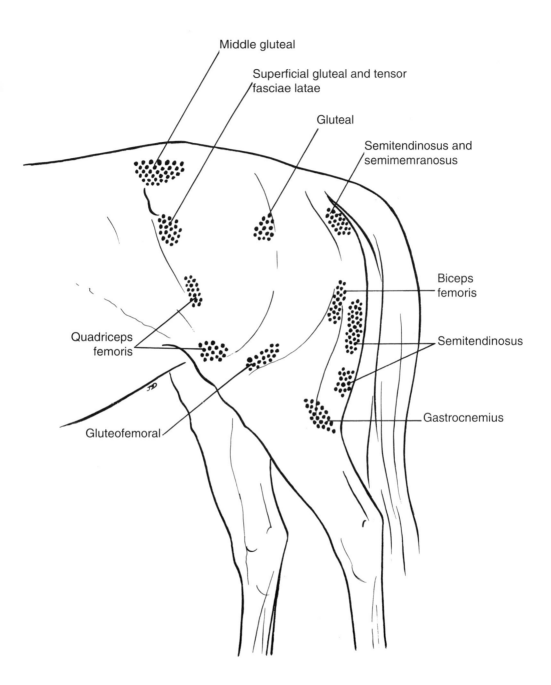

Figure 73 Tension points in the croup and thigh.

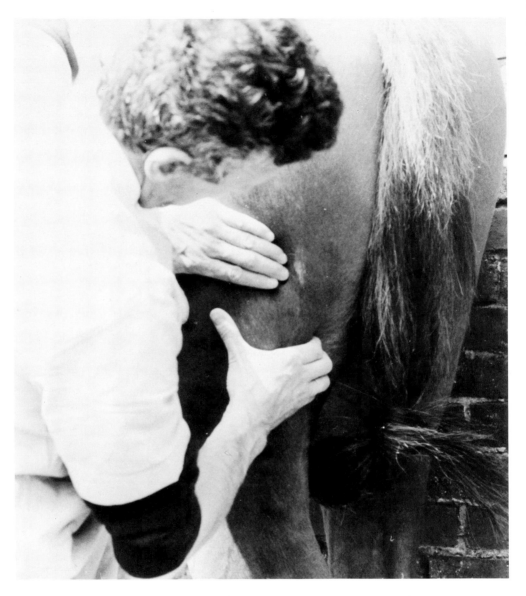

Photo 34 Massage of the caudal muscles in the thigh.

dorso-caudal chain. Pathology and treatment are as for the preceding two muscles. The gluteofemoral is most often affected in the lower third of its muscular body.

(e) Extensors of the stifle (quadriceps femoris and tensor fasciae latae)
Laterally these muscles are arranged as follows:

1. Tensor fasciae latae and vastus lateralis on the deeper level.
2. Rectus femoris and vastus medialis.

Together they work to engage the hindlimb, and form part of the myofascial ventral chain. Lesions most often occur around the kneecap, and are of ligamentary and tendinous origin. The proximal insertion of the tensor fasciae latae is also a vulnerable area.

1. TREATMENT AND RE-EDUCATION

1. Penetrating transversal massage, with petrissage, 15 min.
2. Ultrasound.
3. Iontophoresis applied both inside and outside the area around the kneecap, on the lateral ligaments.
4. Ascents and descents at the walk, with the use of cavalettis.

(f) Gastrocnemius

This is an extensor of the hock and is thus involved in propulsion. In cases of injury, one finds that contractions come from deep within the muscle. In the box the horse lies with the limb gently flexed while resting. It experiences difficulties with support, propulsion and engagement due to the interference with the sliding of the bundles of muscle fibres. The key point is often located at the junction between the tendon and muscle.

1. RE-EDUCATION

1. Treatment is the same as for the muscles described above.
2. Massage is very important to help repair damaged myofibrils and revascularize the muscle. The strokes should be deep and transversal, and be applied to the muscle body and to the musculo-tendinous junction.

5.4 MASSAGE OF THE ACUPUNCTURE POINTS (see Fig. 74)

73   location: small cavity between L6 and S1;
     to treat: dorso-lumbar rheumatism, myositis in the hip muscles.
75   location: 2 measures below 73;
     to treat: fatigue and exhaustion.
110 location: small cavity on the croup, 3 measures down from the top of the spinous process of S2;
     to treat: myositis of the gluteal and caudal ischial muscles, sciatica.
111 location: 2 measures caudal to 110;
     to treat: same problems as 110.
113 location: behind the cord of tensor fasciae latae (TFL), in the angle of the hip at the level of its insertion;
     to treat: same problems as 110 and 111. Lesions of the TFL.
114 location: small cavity anterior to and within the hip joint, at the insertion of the rectus femoris;
     to treat: oedema in the hindlimb, arthrosis in the hip.
115 location: posterior face of the femur;
     to treat: contraction of the muscles in the croup.
117 location: small cavity below the ischial tuberosity;
     to treat: sciatica, myositis in the femoral muscles.

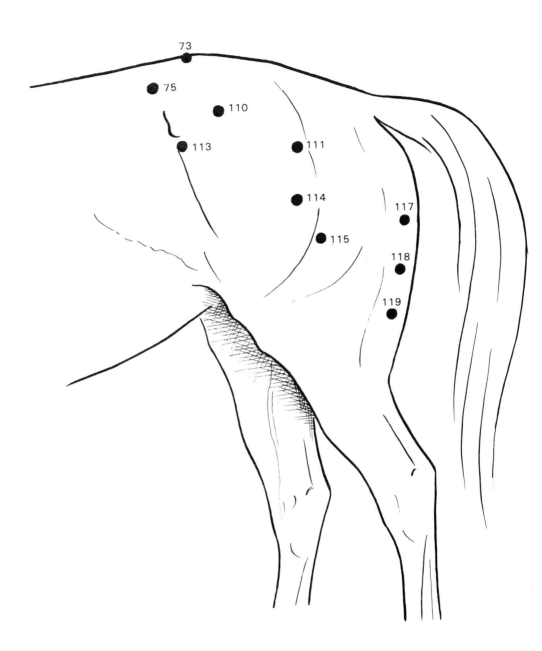

Figure 74 Acupuncture points in the pelvis and thigh.

118   location: small cavity 2 measures below 117;
   to treat: contraction and myositis in the local muscles and tendons.

5.5 FEMOROPATELLAR SYNDROME

As the angle of the knee joint increases during locomotion, the patella can catch on the medial tubercle of the femoral trochlea, causing an impediment. The advice given by R. Barone is as follows:

> "In order to free up the angle of the joint, it is necessary that [the horse] uses a few fibres in the quadriceps femoris to gently raise the kneecap; this will help avoid this check to locomotion. Failure to do so will result in the characteristic catching of the kneecap, during which the limb remains stiff in extension due to fibrous formations around its various joints."

While cases may not get as far as blocking extension, one can be confronted with cases of intermittent catching, which can interfere with the regularity and soundness of the trot. There can also be reactions to this phenomenon in the lumbar region. These are often improved following treatment and femoro-patellar re-education.

5.6 PHYSIOTHERAPY

1. First 3 days, resting in the box.
2. Ultrasound applied to the internal and external collateral ligaments around the kneecap; 12 min on each side. Deep transverse massage on the same ligaments using an anti-inflammatory ointment. Repeat both daily for 10 days.
3. Re-education: going out for walks, interspersed with trotting; limit work on two tracks as well as figures which involve raising the legs. Jumps regulated by cavalettis, preferably at the trot.

5 Preparation of Muscles for Specific kinds of Competition

1. HARNESS RACING

With wheelhorses concentrate on the lumbo-gluteal and caudal muscles. One often finds powerful tensions in the lumbar muscles, usually the gluteus medius and those around the ilium. With leadhorses focus on the lower part of the neck (trapezius and serratus cervicalis) which often suffer particularly badly during long distance racing.

2. OBSTACLE JUMPING

The shoulders should be examined both before and after competition for damage or strain to the muscles involved in 'locking' during landing; these are especially prone to cramps and pain after long competitions, and need to be relaxed if sound functioning is to be restored in time for the next round. The paravertebral muscles (trapezius, rhomboid and erector spinae) and the propulsor muscles in the hindquarters (middle gluteal, gluteobiceps and caudal femoral) should also be examined closely and given appropriate care.

3. DRESSAGE

The pectoral muscles act as a brake on the extension of the arm as it descends; they are involved in simultaneous stretching and braking, and, if inadequately prepared, can be subjected to unexpected elongation. As a result, they are often sensitive and painful and require slow and very gentle treatment using transverse and longitudinal strokes. A further problem is presented by the transverse 'corset' formed by the fibres in the ascending pectoral, which may not provide adequate support and vascular drainage; frequently, metabolic products are not eliminated and thus accumulate, resulting in myalgias which can interfere with amplitude of movement or lead to resistance.

One should also treat the following areas:

1. Shoulders (involved in extensions).
2. Brachiocephalic (involved in extensions).
3. Erector spinae, middle gluteal, gluteobiceps, caudal femoral muscles.
4. Stifle – carefully apply deep transverse massage, using an anti-inflammatory ointment; for delicate horses treatment should be administered 8 days in every month.

Index